Contents

Preface to the First Edition   v

Preface to the Second Edition   vii

List of Authors   ix

1   The Nature of General Practice   1
Michael Drury

2   The Structure of General Practice   6
Michael Drury

3   Training the Primary Care Team   15
Norman Ellis

4   The Nature of Management and Administration   21
Roderick Martin

5   The Role of the Practice Manager   37
Andrew Proctor

6   Personnel Management of Practice Staff   51
Brian Willey

7   Communication, Motivation and Teamwork   83
Michael Hamilton

8   Health and Safety in the Surgery   109
Norman Ellis

9   Quality and its Measurement   117
Douglas Fleming

10   Audit and the Practice Manager   130
Michael Drury

11   Managing Money   138
John Dean

12   Prescribing   187
David Clegg

13   The GP Fund-holding Initiative   191
John Dean

14   Managing Patients   199
John Hasler and Merrill Whalen

Index   232

The New Practice Manager

EDITED BY

MICHAEL DRURY

SECOND EDITION

RADCLIFFE MEDICAL PRESS
OXFORD

First published 1990
Reprinted 1990
Reprinted 1991
Second Edition 1991
Reprinted 1992

British Library Cataloguing in Publication Data
Drury, Michael
    The new practice manager.
    1. Great Britain. General practice. Management
    I. Title
    362.1'72'068

ISBN 1 870905 41 5

Typeset by Advance Typesetting Ltd, Oxfordshire
Printed and bound in Great Britain by
Billing & Sons Ltd, Worcester

Preface to the First Edition

THIS book is written for practice managers and senior receptionists. Whilst it will stand on its own, it is designed to accompany Practice Manager Development, a course in which a group of practice managers (and sometimes doctors) learn together and from each other. Whilst nearly all group practices now have a practice manager their experience and skills are very varied. Some, probably the majority, have been promoted within the practice from receptionist and have learnt and developed as time has passed. These have very often had little opportunity to learn outside the practice, little chance to get support and education from their peer group and it has been difficult to introduce modern management skills from different business areas. A few have come from outside with previous management training but have had to learn the medical component of their job the hard way. This book is designed primarily for the former group but we hope that any practice manager would be helped by it.

The authors have been drawn from outside disciplines and from the medical world in an attempt to get the balance right; the book therefore covers both concepts and practical issues. Managers are concerned with people, equipment and money and the management of all these aspects of general practice is considered.

Not all practice managers are female but for the sake of continuity we have written as if they are and as if the doctors are male. We hope this device will not offend others.

We are grateful to Drs Fleming, Oldroyd, Ridsdill-Smith, Taylor, Pike and Steel who, sometimes with their practice managers, advised on the content of the book. We are also grateful to a large number of secretaries who have helped. Finally, our thanks go to Andrew Bax and Kate Martin at Radcliffe Medical Press and to Ciba-Geigy Pharmaceuticals whose financial help made publication possible.

Professor Sir Michael Drury
Department of General Practice
University of Birmingham

November 1989

Preface to the Second Edition

THE wide acceptance of the first edition of this book has been responsible for the need to reprint it during its first year. Further demand has given an opportunity to produce a Second Edition and to add some new sections, keeping it thoroughly up to date with the rapid changes in the health service. In particular, sections have been added to cover audit, practice prescribing budgets and fund holding. We have also taken the opportunity to make alterations to those sections covering communication, motivation and teamwork as well as revising most other chapters. All concerned in this new edition recognize the importance of the role of practice managers in today's health service and hope that this book will help them with their tasks and add to the satisfaction they obtain.

I would like to acknowledge the help of David Clegg and Michael Hamilton, who have joined our team of contributors for this edition, and of Janice Downing and Pauline Shepherd, who advised in its preparation.

Professor Sir Michael Drury
Department of General Practice
University of Birmingham

May 1991

List of Authors

Dr David Clegg has recently retired as senior partner in a large South East Staffordshire Group Practice after 32 years. For 15 years he was Associate Adviser in General Practice in the West Midlands, with a particular interest in education for general practice. He is now part-time Medical Adviser to Wolverhampton FHSA.

John Dean is Director of Medical Services in Pannell Kerr Forster's Home Counties area. He has specialized in this field for over 15 years and is accepted as a leading authority on the subject. He writes extensively for the medical and dental journals; and has been a contributor on the Institute of Chartered Accountants course and is a co-author of a recently published guide to GPs' pensions. His book *Making Sense of Practice Finance* was published during 1990.

Professor Sir Michael Drury has been in general practice in Bromsgrove since 1953. He is Professor of General Practice in Birmingham and a past President of the Royal College of General Practitioners. He has researched and written widely about practice organization and has been deeply involved in establishing receptionist and practice nurse training programmes.

Norman Ellis is Under Secretary of the British Medical Association, the head of the BMA Division which looks after general practice and provides the secretariat of the General Medical Services Committee. Author of *Employing Staff*, a British Medical Journal publication and a frequent contributor to the medical press on practice management and medico-political subjects.

Dr Douglas Fleming graduated in 1959 and is now a senior partner in a group of five principals working in Birmingham. He has been associated with the Birmingham Research Unit of the Royal College of General Practitioners for 25 years and has had considerable involvement in the Weekly Return Service, National Morbidity Studies and more recently in the development of Practice Activity Analysis.

Michael Hamilton has worked in personnel and GP administration in the NHS in Edinburgh for 15 years. He lectures in health services management, practice management, primary health care and social policy; and is an examiner for the Institute of Health Services Management. He writes for Radcliffe Medical Press on Practice Manager Development and is currently also involved in NHS developments of new GP computer systems.

Dr John Hasler has been a general practitioner in South Oxfordshire since 1966 and Regional Postgraduate Adviser in General Practice for the Oxford Region since 1972. He is past Honorary Secretary and Chairman of the Council of the Royal College of General Practitioners, and has written extensively in the general practice literature.

Roderick Martin, Fellow in Management, Templeton College, Oxford since 1988. Previously Professor of Industrial Sociology at Imperial College, University of London and Fellow of Trinity College, Oxford. His particular interests include the effects of new technology on work.

Dr Andrew Proctor is a general practitioner in Lincolnshire. He has been a general practitioner in Central Manchester and Bury and was formerly Lecturer in General Practice at the University of Manchester.

Merrill Whalen is Training Adviser with Ross Hall AMI Hospital, Glasgow. Formerly she was a practice manager in Edinburgh, has written extensively on management in the medical press, and frequently lectures on courses. Her particular interest is the training of practice staff and she was heavily involved in the development of Practice Receptionist Programme.

Brian Willey is a Senior Lecturer at Kingston Polytechnic. He currently teaches industrial relations and employment law, and previously worked in reseach and education for a large union.

1 The Nature of General Practice

THIS chapter aims to explore the philosophy of general practice. What are its objectives? What is the nature of the problems that it faces and what solutions does it offer? These questions are important ones for the practice manager to address because she will have to subscribe to that philosophy if she is to make the most of her contribution to patient care.

Everyone who considers himself or herself to be ill needs a point of first contact with a physician which allows entry into the health care system. This frontline medical care is known as 'primary care' in contrast to that of 'secondary care' which is specialized and more sophisticated than that handled in primary care and to which access is usually gained only after being filtered or sorted within primary care. Most countries have some such system but whereas in the UK it is called 'general practice' in other countries it may be 'family practice', 'primary medical care' or 'primary health care'. Whatever the title it has certain characteristics above and beyond being a point of first contact.

1 *The problems presented are undifferentiated.* People do not have to make decisions about the nature of their problem, only that they have one and that it is probably concerned with their health. They do not have to decide whether their chest pain is due to their heart, in which case they would need the advice of a cardiologist or that it may be indigestion and a stomach specialist would be more appropriate. Their problems may be life-threatening or they may be trivial. Furthermore it is the patient's perception of this which is relevant, not the receptionist's, the manager's or the doctor's, so access to care has to be as unrestricted as possible. This is a very important idea to grasp because it clearly shapes how we behave to patients, what we say and the sort of systems that we organize. General practice has to be 'comprehensive'.

2 *Care is offered to the family group.* The fact that problems are undifferentiated and that any age may attend obviously allows all members of the family to be seen but the concept embraced is wider than this. All illness should be regarded as potentially 'family illness'. It is clear that, say, marital disharmony will affect the husband and wife and almost certainly have an impact on children, grandparents and even brothers and sisters whose affections can be stressed. It is not so obvious that, say, a duodenal ulcer can affect the family but the diet, the need for rest and quiet, the effect upon temper, holidays, sexual relationships can all be factors in the management.

Another perspective of the significance of family care is the need to explore and make the best of this opportunity within a consultation. The spouse who accompanies the patient is expressing concern and caring and needs to be considered. The act of immunizing a child is more than giving an injection, it is an opportunity to establish a relationship with a mother, to discuss feeding, growth, education and behaviour at a time when the mother is very receptive to these ideas.

3 *Care is continuous*. Much care is episodic. A patient may come once with a boil, take advice, perhaps receive a prescription and have urine tested for glycosuria and then leave, but most care is prolonged for most illness is chronic or recurrent. Tables 1.1, 1.2 and 1.3 show the approximate frequency with which common and rare problems may be seen in a practice of 10 000 persons and it will be noted that chronic disease is a longer list and represents several consultations for that condition each year. The right-hand figure gives the number of persons consulting per year from a list of 10 000 patients.

Table 1.1 Minor conditions.

Tonsillitis	400
Acute otitis media	350
Cystitis	200
Back pain	200
Migraine	120
Hay fever	100

Table 1.2 Acute major conditions.

Acute chest infection	200
Coronary thromboses	30
Acute appendix	20
Stroke	20
All cancers	20

Nearly all chronic disease is now treated within the community. Some, such as hypertension, are nearly always treated within general practice, but other problems may sometimes be treated by other agencies, specialists, hospitals, private sources and so on. However, because primary care is continuous the record card is the only repository of all medical information and the responsibility for manipulating and co-ordinating care across boundaries, in short 'managing', is the task of general practice. That is why we have a referral system and why all the letters eventually return from the periphery to the centre of the web. The patient with a stroke may be seen at the hospital, or even admitted for a while, but the responsibility for continuity of care, for organizing transport, meals-on-wheels, physiotherapy or chiropody is ultimately that of general practice although, of course, it is often convenient to delegate it to others. Again the implications of this concept are great and the practice team has a vital role in co-ordinating good quality care. Certainly patients see this as a most important function and breakdown as a fearful addition to existing problems of ill health.

Table 1.3 Some chronic disease in general practice: annual person consulting rates.

	Annual persons consulting per 10 000 patients
High blood pressure	1000
Chronic rheumatism, arthritis	400
Chronic mental	400
Ischaemic heart disease	200
Obesity	200
All cancers	120
Asthma	120
Diabetes	120
Strokes	80
Epilepsy	40
Multiple sclerosis	12

From: *N.H.S. Data Book*, eds Fry, J., Brooks, D. & McColl, I. M.T. Press Ltd. (1984).

It also has very important implications for management in terms of activity. Letters arrive from hospitals asking us to prescribe a drug, arrange an investigation or review after a period of time and that action has to be taken otherwise the patient may suffer, the hospital be given extra work or even litigation ensue.

Continuity of care has one other aspect that must be considered here. Care given by a variety of people can soon become fragmented and confusing for the patient. It needs some skill directed to the problem to enable one person, or as few people as necessary to become involved. For example a patient dying at home needs to be cared for by their nurse and their doctor. At the same time cover by other informed people is necessary when the key people cannot be there.

4 *Care includes disease prevention and health promotion.* One of the most profound shifts in the philosophy of general practice in the past few years has been the change from a 'reactive' pattern of working to a 'pro-active' one. The best simile is that provided by the fire brigade. Their 'reactive' pattern of work is to sally forth at high speed in response to a call

that your house is on fire. Their 'pro-active' work involves calling to advise on safety precautions, fire-proof doors, smoke detectors, etc. that might prevent a catastrophe. Similarly, in general practice, when a family registers with the practice they are saying 'please be there when we want you' but they are also saying 'please stop us suffering from illness that can be avoided'. Of course patients are autonomous; they are at liberty to decline, without fear of causing offence, the advice that is offered, but it is the responsibility of the health professional to make certain that they are informed, and understand the issues. A general practice has a responsibility for each individual patient but it has also a wider responsibility to its whole population. We need to protect from infectious disease by immunizing the well; to detect early illness by measuring blood pressure, screening for cancer of the cervix or high blood cholesterol and to promote good health by considering diet, smoking, alcohol intake, exercise and relaxation in well people.

Why us and not someone else you may ask? We have two great assets on our side. Firstly most people see a doctor regularly. Every year nearly 70% of the people on our list will attend the surgery; by the end of two years that figure will have risen to 80% and by a further year to 90%. That provides a tremendous chance for opportunistic screening or advice giving, but if it is to be effective every person in the team needs to be alert to that chance. Secondly patients are 'switched on' to health concerns when they consult so health education makes a great impact at this time. Fear is a great force towards taking action to prevent ill health.

5 *Care attends to the whole person.* Wholism has become something of a cliché in the past few years and the concept has been grasped by others who have often accused the medical profession of being so disease-centred—'he was only interested in my liver'—that they ignored the person outside the disease. There is some justification in this view in some of our behaviour but we have moved progressively further towards a much more rounded approach. We are now comfortable with this and have encapsulated the concept by constructing diagnoses or management plans in interlocking areas of physical, psychological and social factors.

Clearly at times, or with particular diseases one of these components is predominant. A young man with a fractured tibia has a largely physical problem, but even here there may be anxiety about his ability to play football in the future that constitutes a major worry and problems with his work of a social nature. If these are not considered he may rightly feel incompletely cared for. In other situations, such as malignant disease or depression other areas become predominant but they are all always there. Administration needs to grasp this idea if it is to recognize the different reasons for seeking care and the different patterns of behaviour of those who come.

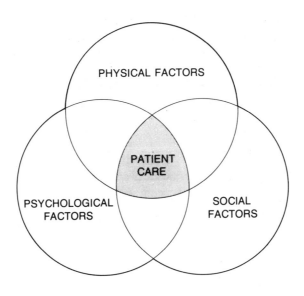

Figure 1.1

In 1969 the Royal College of General Practitioners published a job definition of the general practitioner and it is as true today as when it was first written.

Job definition

'The general practitioner is a doctor who provides personal, primary and continuing medical care to individuals and families. He may attend his patients in their homes, in his consulting-room or sometimes in hospital. He accepts the responsibility for making an initial decision on every problem his patient may present to him, consulting with specialists when he thinks it appropriate to do so. He will usually work in a group with other general practitioners, from premises that are built or modified for the purpose, with the help of paramedical colleagues, adequate secretarial staff and all the equipment which is necessary. Even if he is in single-handed practice, he will work in a team and delegate when necessary. His diagnoses will be composed in physical, psychological and social terms. He will intervene educationally, preventively and therapeutically to promote his patient's health.'

(From p.1 of *The Future General Practitioner*, Royal College of General Practitioners, 1972.)

2 The Structure of General Practice

MOST practice managers will already have a clear understanding of the structure of the practice within which they work so this chapter will not describe this but will concentrate, rather, on the ideas behind the structure and the way it is changing and will seek to explore some of the philosophy behind these changes. We shall describe briefly some of the outside organizations with which general practice relates as the new functions and structure of these may be less well-known to practice managers.

The general practitioner (GP) has a different relationship with the health service to that of doctors working in hospitals. He is not an employee of the health service as they are but an independent contractor. This is an important difference which shapes and directs the way in which general practice is managed and develops. To understand the concept of 'independent contractor status' it is helpful to use an analogy from the construction industry. The builder who has the task of developing a housing estate directly employs a number of workers who labour, lay bricks and work with timber. He also needs electricity put into these houses—wiring, plugs, cooker points and so on—but he does not directly employ electricians so he gives a contract to a firm of electricians to do this, specifying what is required and how much he will pay for the completed job but he leaves the details of the work to the 'independent' firm to arrange and only requires a satisfactory job to be done within the time and price agreed by the firm who is thus an 'independent contractor'. In this same way the GP has a contract to supply services to patients who are registered by the FHSA as on his list. It is his responsibility to provide the premises, time, equipment and systems required to do a proper job. There is considerable flexibility about how and where he does this providing that it is done within the broad guidelines of the contract.

An independent contractor is therefore a self-employed person who has entered into a contract for services with another party. This contract *for* services is fundamentally different from a contract *of* services, which governs employee – employer relationships and is explained in greater detail in *Making Sense of the New Contract* ed. J. Chisholm, Radcliffe Medical Press, Oxford (1990), but it is essentially a difference in the amount of control that exists.

The GP then is not an employee of the Family Health Services Authority (FHSA). If he makes a mistake the responsibility is his, not that of the FHSA. If he had been an employee then the employer, the FHSA, would also have been responsible if a mistake was made. Of course the contract agreed between the two parties is much more explicit than this and contains rules about hours of work and access by patients, about the standards of premises and where doctors may live, but much of the work is bound by general statements, such as 'a doctor shall render his patients all necessary and appropriate personal services of the type usually provided by general practitioners', or 'shall keep adequate records of the illnesses and treatment of his patient on forms supplied to him for the purpose by the Authority', or 'shall do so at his premises or, if the condition of the patient so requires, elsewhere in his practice area', etc. It will be noted at once that the use of words and phrases such as 'necessary and appropriate', 'adequate' and so on raise issues of what is adequate or necessary and by whom it is so judged.

The functions of the previous Family Practitioner Committee was mainly to administer the contract with doctors (and dentists, opticians and pharmacists) and to maintain the register of patients, and it had nearly half of its members drawn from professional bodies. With the new FHSAs this has changed. Why has this change been proposed? The answer lies partly within the concept of the independent contractor. The advantage of this system is, primarily, its flexibility. As practices can control their own methods and systems for providing care a good deal of variation occurs depending on local differences. Populations, patients, staff, buildings and local geography are all different and what suits one practice may not suit others. The potential disadvantage is that the variation may become too great. There may be such a variation that unacceptable standards are allowed to exist. The FHSA has the responsibilities of planning, developing and managing the services provided by general medical practitioners, general dental practitioners, retail pharmacists and opticians. In England there are 90 FHSAs relating to 14 Regional Health Authorities (RHAs). The eight FHSAs in Wales relate to the Welsh Office, whereas in Scotland there are 15 Health Boards responsible for hospital, community and family health services and in Northern Ireland four Health & Social Services Boards (see Fig. 2.1).

The FHSAs in England look after populations ranging between 130 000 and 1 600 000. Nearly 40 of these share a boundary with a single District Health Authority (DHA) but the remainder relate to between two and seven DHAs. The Chairman of each FHSA is appointed by the Secretary of State. There are also five lay non-executive members appointed by the RHA and this group appoints the General Manager. The FHSA is completed by four other executive members, a GP, a dentist, a pharmacist and a community nurse, works as a corporate body and is accountable, in England, to the RHA.

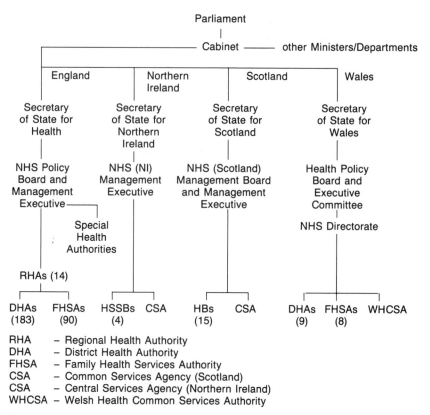

RHA   – Regional Health Authority
DHA   – District Health Authority
FHSA   – Family Health Services Authority
CSA   – Common Services Agency (Scotland)
CSA   – Central Services Agency (Northern Ireland)
WHCSA – Welsh Health Common Services Authority

Figure 2.1   Diagram (simplified) of the management organization of the NHS in 1991 – from Parliament to health authority level.

The functions of the FHSA, in relationship to general practice, are to:

- manage the contracts of GPs;
- pay GPs;
- provide information to the public;
- deal with complaints made by patients;
- assess the health needs of the population;
- develop services that are effective and efficient.

The last two of these functions are the ones that really mark the change from the past and in order to carry them out new tasks have arisen. There will need to be a much larger base of information held by the authority and developed in relation to DHAs and local authorities. For example, in planning services for children the registers of children born in the district and those who move into the district will need to be combined and the resources involved in, say, immunization, from all three authorities will need to be co-ordinated. There are new tasks associated with carrying out consumer surveys, supporting continuing education for the staff in practices, encouraging medical audit, monitoring indicative prescribing amounts, and developing with RHAs fund-holding practices. There are also the old tasks of inspecting premises, approving surgery locations and hours of availability, monitoring deputizing services and dealing with complaints.

District Health Authorities (DHAs)

The DHA is responsible for purchasing hospital and community health services for the population in its area. It is an employer of staff, nurses, porters, cooks and cleaners as well as junior doctors, it has to run services provided by the hospitals to in-patients and out-patients, laboratory services and so on. The duties relating to the community services which, whilst they may account for only a small part of the budget, are very important. These include home nursing, midwifery and health visiting services and often those supplied to certain groups of people for, say, family planning and paediatric surveillance in clinics, school health services, etc. It is the fact that different authorities, FHSAs and DHAs for instance, are responsible for many of the same services that leads to confusion and conflict.

As we have seen there is an increased need for the various authorities to work together. One example of this is the Child Health Surveillance Programme requiring the co-operation of FHSA services, DHA services and local authority and school services. Others are the cervical cytology programme and services for the care of the aged. The implications of this for practice managers are obvious and important. The exchange of information by the accurate completion of forms and, increasingly, with the aid of computers allows much more reliable care to be provided to the population of the practice.

The boundary between hospital services and community services is, in any case somewhat artificial. Patients do not respect it and they move backwards and forwards, as do specimens, forms and sometimes doctors. Perhaps the difficulties that exist will be alleviated by the fact that from now on FHSAs and DHAs will both be responsible to RHAs making co-operation between them potentially more easy.

In England there are 14 RHAs (four within London and ten outside) and each contains a number of Districts. There are 189 DHAs and the populations served by them range from 89 000 (Rugby) to 860 000 (Leicestershire). They contain either a single District General Hospital or several hospitals and between 50 and 400 GPs who mainly relate to these hospitals. In Wales there are nine districts, Scotland has 15 Health Boards and Northern Ireland a structure of four Health & Social Services Boards with 36 'units' below them.

Each DHA has a Chairman appointed by the Secretary of State, five non-executive members appointed by the RHA and five executive members. The General Manager and the Chief Finance Officers are ex-officio executive members.

The functions of the DHA are:

- purchasing services;
- managing services;
- assessing needs for health care;
- public health responsibilities.

Local Medical Committees (LMCs)

Prior to 1990 nearly half the members of the Family Practitioner Committee were drawn from the professional organizations and eight came from the Local Medical Committee (LMC). In future there is to be one GP on the FHSA, probably from the LMC. This obviously suggests a different relationship between the two organizations. Members of the LMC are elected by all the GPs in an area on a constituency basis so it is a powerful way in which opinions can be sought. Until recently there has been a statutory requirement for the FHSA to consult LMCs on a variety of issues, but it is uncertain how this relationship will operate in future. It is certain, however, that the FHSA will need to consult widely with the professional bodies in its management role for unless agreement can be reached on the way the services should be developed, progress and patient care will be harmed. There are likely to be new lines of communication developed. One example of this will be within the Medical Audit Advisory Groups to be set up by each FHSA for scrutiny of the quality of clinical service provided. This is a professional matter relying on clinical judgments, but to be successful it will need managerial input. The Group has to be serviced and the FHSA is in possession of data that is essential for clinical audit. We shall see later in this book how the practice manager has important tasks in relationship to audit. When the audit spreads more widely than the practice the LMC might well become involved.

The LMC is a very important source of information for the individual practitioner or the practice. It is perhaps the first point to which a doctor turns when seeking advice about the meaning of the regulations which govern his or her terms of service. For the past 23 years the Red Book (the Statement of Fees and Allowances) has set out the basis on which GPs are paid and practices financed. Doctors and practice managers need to master this system and understand what the regulations mean.*

---

*Further information can be obtained from *Making Sense of the New Contract*, ed. J. Chisholm. Radcliffe Medical Press, Oxford (1990).

Negotiations with, and advice given to, the Government concerning general practice comes mainly from a standing committee of the BMA called the General Medical Services Committee (GMSC). Whilst this is not controlled by the LMCs it takes advice from them through an annual meeting of representation of all LMCs in the country.

Some hospitals and similar units have been established as self-governing units within the NHS. They are managed by boards of directors and are not responsible to DHAs or RHAs but directly to the Secretary of State. They earn their income by selling services to health authorities, GP fund holders or other purchasers and are responsible for both quality and quantity of service. They can determine their own management structure, employ staff, borrow money and act with greater freedom than DHAs. They are an experiment designed to devolve power and decisions down to managers, doctors, nurses and other staff.

Local Authorities

The relationship between social conditions and medical problems is so intertwined that the impact upon medical care of the presence or absence of social services provided by the local authority is profound. Furthermore most issues relating to environmental health, such as the control of infection, are their responsibility as well.

The practice's first contact with the Social Services Department is usually by telephone and is dealt with by a duty social worker. He or she will, if the problem cannot be dealt with at this level, usually refer it to one of the Divisions for attention. With the ageing of the general population the need for both residential care and domiciliary services has increased and the government has now accepted the principle that Local Authorities are to be responsible for all residential care of the elderly and handicapped. The emphasis is, however, on maintaining people in their own homes for as long as possible and this means that GPs will have to play a bigger part in assessing care for the elderly and will be responsible for notifying the Local Authorities of their patients' needs for non-health care. This is related to the requirement for the over-75s to be seen at least once annually.

The history of communication between medical services and social services is generally poor and often somewhat antagonistic. When this occurs it is always the patient that suffers so anything to improve matters that can be done by a practice will help. Part of the trouble is that of different time scales, doctors who are often called in urgently when a crisis occurs need an urgent service whereas social workers have competing demands that take time to meet. Another part of the problem is caused by

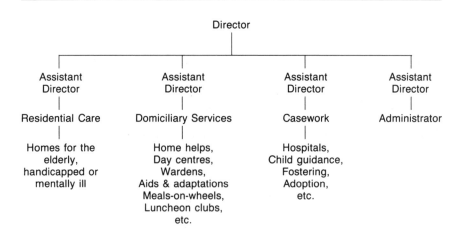

Figure 2.2 The organization of a typical Social Services Department.

a failure on both sides to understand the nature of the other's task and the constraints within which people operate. Where social workers are attached to practices most of these difficulties seem to melt away.

Community Health Councils (CHCs)

These are present in each of the 189 Health Districts in England and the 9 Health Districts in Wales. In Scotland, Local Health Councils (LHCs) perform the same functions. CHCs were set up in 1974 to provide a stronger consumer voice within the service and they are required to assess the adequacy of local services from the user's viewpoint. They have a right to be informed about planning and operation of services, to be consulted if a hospital is to be closed and to visit NHS hospitals and institutions. They have access to DHAs and their senior officers and the DHA is required to publish replies describing action taken on issues raised in the CHC's annual report.

They normally have about 20 members, half appointed by the Local Authority, one third by voluntary organizations and the remainder by the RHA. They do not have a right to visit GP's premises although they do take up issues relating to primary care with the FHSA. In some respects they are regarded as 'toothless tigers' but many practices recognize them as an important source of consumer opinion and are anxious to develop better communication with them and to invite them to visit practices and discuss matters with practice staff.

They have rights to:

- access to some NHS premises;
- inclusion in the consultation process when there are substantial changes in the services;
- send observers to DHA and FHSA meetings;
- obtain some information from NHS authorities.

They publish an annual report which is discussed by FHSAs and DHAs.

Trends in the change of practice

In the first 40 years of the NHS general practice has much enlarged and strengthened. We do not know if change will continue in the same direction but it is worth noting briefly the major changes that have occurred.

The number of GPs has greatly increased from about 18 000 in 1949 to over 30 000 in 1989. Whilst the population has also increased over this period it has meant that the average number of patients for whom a GP is responsible has dropped from over 2 500 to under 2 000. At the same time the average number of consultations that each patient makes with each GP has decreased slightly and is now about 4.4 per annum for females and 3.3 per annum for males. The rate is highest at the two extremes of age but these trends have allowed the average length of a consultation to grow from four minutes to nearly nine minutes and this permits much more to be done.

In 1949 over 80% of GPs were in single-handed practice. Today more than 80% are in partnership and the size of groups is gradually increasing. Patients are more mobile and telephone usage is much higher so close proximity to the doctor's surgery is less important. The advantages of group practice should include:

- greater sharing of costs;
- ability to use a wider range of equipment;
- ability to employ a wider range of staff;
- greater choice for patients;
- less professional isolation for doctors and staff.

All principals in general practice are now fully trained and over 1 000 practices are designated training practices. (The practice manager in such a practice should familiarize herself with the structure and objectives of the training programme.) The number of female doctors is increasing and half the output of a medical school is now female. During the 1960s there was a large intake of new doctors by immigration. This is now smaller but the new regulations within the EEC may alter this situation.

There has been a major rehousing of general practice to accommodate group practice and this has also allowed a great expansion of practice staff from a few hundred in 1949 to about 40 000 whole time equivalents in 1989. There have been many factors influencing these trends. Some are financial (they can be more cost-effective), some are clinical (they can provide better care), and some have to do with changing values of patients and doctors who, say, want off-duty rotas, appointment systems, accommodation for wheelchairs, babies and so on. Whatever the reasons the whole structure is much more complex and this is the *raison d'etre* for practice management and practice managers.

3 Training the Primary Care Team

THE staff are probably the most important asset in general practice, and GPs owe it to them and to themselves to ensure that they are able to work to the best of their capabilities. Although it seems obvious that a new employee should be trained and properly introduced into the work of the practice, this vital task is often neglected or forgotten by GPs. If adequate induction and training are not provided, any employer can put himself seriously at risk if it subsequently proves necessary to take disciplinary action: this omission can provide the employee with an effective defence against any criticism of the standard of her performance or behaviour. The term 'induction' is widely used to describe the process of training and education provided for a new employee, and although it may be another unwelcome example of technical jargon, for once the use of such a term helps because it does convey the precise meaning intended.

If considerable time and resources have been devoted to selecting capable staff, this could be wasted if induction and training are not provided, enabling them to become familiar with the working arrangements of the practice and to work effectively.

Why 'induction' is so important

Any employer will want the new employee to settle into the working arrangements of the practice as quickly as possible. To achieve this the GP and his colleagues will need to help her to become familiar with many aspects of the practice and its day-to-day work, to know the wide range of outside contacts that will become part of her job; the FHSA, other GP practices, local hospitals, the deputizing service, Social Services Department, community nursing services, etc. Most important of all, she will need to be helped and guided in getting to grips with the job itself. Only when the new employee begins to feel reasonably competent in the job can she achieve personal satisfaction from contributing effectively to the work of the practice.

Much of this knowledge will be acquired gradually without any formal training, 'sitting next to Nellie'. Indeed, if formalized training is provided too early, this will be largely wasted and the new recruit will be left confused rather than informed. Many of us will recall from personal experience laborious and detailed induction talks of this kind which singularly failed to impart any lasting knowledge. Nothing is worse than too much information being given too soon.

When a new employee starts work she will be anxious about some aspects of the new job. She is simultaneously having to become acquainted with a new environment, new tasks, new colleagues and a new boss. If the new employee is helped to settle in as early as possible, she is not only being shown the courtesy and consideration that may be reasonably expected, it is also helping to make the practice run smoothly. Induction is just as important in a small business as in any large organization which runs formal training courses, and need not be costly in time and resources. However, if it is not done, the consequences may be very costly indeed.

A new employee cannot be expected to be able to fulfil the demands of her job until she has settled into the practice. She has an initial (and hopefully steep) learning curve to climb and she will be unable to respond effectively and quickly. The time lag before a satisfactory performance is achieved is likely to be greatly increased if you make no arrangements for induction. Important instructions are more likely to be forgotten and misunderstood, and vital procedures may be ignored. The new employee's early enthusiasm may wane before she feels settled, and she may become disillusioned and even consider leaving. This disenchantment will reduce effectiveness and can even cause difficulties within the practice training. By ensuring that the induction programme is effective many of these problems can be prevented.

When does induction start?

Surprisingly enough, the induction process actually starts when prospective employees are being interviewed. All applicants who are interviewed for a vacancy in a practice should learn something about how it is run. The interviewee should have acquired an initial impression of her prospective colleagues when shown around the surgery and introduced to the staff. After being selected for the post, it may be helpful to invite the prospective employee to come back to meet her future colleagues informally before she is formally offered the job and accepts it. In the small and tight-knit community of the primary health care team it is vital that all its members are compatible and conflicts of personality are avoided.

The employer should ensure that the new employee is made to feel welcome on her very first day; the practice manager should make a special effort, at this time, to give the newcomer her full attention. It is common practice to ask new recruits to start at a later time on the first day and, in general practice it may be advisable to arrange the arrival time after morning surgery has ended; this allows the practice manager to give the new employee undivided attention. For a new recruit to arrive at, say, 8.30 or 9.00 a.m. on a Monday morning, and to sit around for two hours watching others working hard can be disarming and dispiriting.

The induction programme may last several days, or even weeks; in practice it should not take long to complete. Whatever time span is chosen, it must be comprehensive. It is important to recognize that a new employee can only absorb a limited amount of information at a time, but also on the other hand, as she becomes more settled in the practice the more difficult it becomes to find time for training.

A new employee must be allowed sufficient time to become confident in the job. In general practice, surgery staff often face a continuous and high pressure of work throughout the day; in this respect the new employee is likely to experience far greater pressure than in any previous job. For this reason it is essential that she is able to become gradually accustomed to the new working pattern.

Prepare a checklist for your induction plan

Induction training is likely to be informal, but nevertheless it should follow a definite plan. Often the plan is written down in the form of a checklist to ensure that all stages are covered and accounted for (*see* Box 3.1). The practice manager should be closely involved in preparing this plan and implementing it. It is likely that much of the induction training will be undertaken by the practice manager and other experienced members of the team. Nevertheless, although the specific tasks may be delegated, it is advisable for one of the partners to be the responsible person to whom the manager reports on training matters. In any case, one partner should certainly take a personal interest in the new employee and make sure that satisfactory working relationships with the doctors are developed. To a new employee, particularly a young person, the doctors themselves can appear to be formidable and unapproachable. This direct contact between a partner and the new employee should help to ensure that the practice's methods and objectives are not diluted or misunderstood, and may even offer even greater insight into the day-to-day running of the practice.

Box 3.1: Example of an induction checklist

First day at work

- layout of the surgery:
  cloakroom and toilet facilities
  first-aid provision
  'mess' arrangements

- the job (refer to job description as appropriate)
  new entrant's own job
  supervision arrangements
  colleagues (including introductions to partners)
  standard of work expected

Second day at work

- explaining the conditions of employment
  (refer to employment contract as appropriate)
  hours of work
  lunch and tea breaks
  periods of notice
  timekeeping
  method of paying salary
  income tax and national insurance and any other deductions
  holidays
  sick leave, medical statement and rules, for example
    arrangements for reporting absences
  pension scheme

Third day at work

- the practice:
  range of services to patients
  organization of practice
  relations with other bodies and organizations
  brief history and outline of future developments

During the induction programme a new recruit will need to listen to her colleagues explaining their work and how the surgery runs, and to watch the pattern of work. She should be encouraged to ask questions, however basic or simple. Reference may also be made to written statement of the terms and conditions of employment and her job description when explaining how the practice is organized and how her job fits in.

As a broad guide to the time involved, induction training could take a half day during the first day of week, perhaps one or two hours on each of the remaining days during the first week, and then at least one or two hours each week during the first month.

All recruits and promotees need induction

Although every new member of staff will need some induction training, certain groups of people may well acquire special help and advice. Many employers fail to provide any induction for employees who are either transferred between jobs or promoted. Though this may not be necessary, you should never assume that a competent receptionist or secretary will immediately be transformed into an effective practice manager on promotion. Promotions within a small organization, such as a practice, can cause difficulties if the newly promoted employee is not given advice and assistance. It is unreasonable to expect someone readily to assume the authority and responsibilities of a manager in relation to former colleagues who were previously her 'equals'. Promotion to a supervisory position involves a large increase in responsibility, and this is difficult enough to cope with, without the added problem of doing so among colleagues. If the promotion is to be successful for all concerned, a partner should take on the responsibility of regularly advising and assisting the promotee.

Similarly, it should never be assumed that a new recruit from a similar position in a neighbouring practice will easily fit into another practice. Indeed, a particular effort may be required to retrain this person so that she understands and applies the method and philosophy of the new practice rather than those of her previous employer. New recruits from other practices may have firmly held preconceptions about how the job should be done which are at odds with the arrangements applying to the new job.

Other groups who need help include school leavers and young people without previous work experience. They often need sympathetic but firm assistance in getting to grips with the discipline of a full-time job; punctuality, reliability, consistency, and the usual courtesies of a working environment are particular points to watch. Women returning to employment after a gap of several years can experience special difficulty in regaining confidence. Also special help may be needed for the new employee if she is disabled or from a minority ethnic group.

Who should do the training?

Several people may be involved in the induction training. However, one person should be given overall responsibility for the task and in most practices this will be the practice manager or supervisor. In any case, the practice manager will have the most direct interest in ensuring that the new recruit settles in easily and is soon able to work as an effective member of the team. If the induction is being provided for a receptionist or secretary, the practice manager or another experienced employee will be best equipped to give the initial training. They will know the new employee's job and be directly accessible for advice and assistance. At the same time the new employee should know who to look to for this help.

An essential task which is often forgotten

Induction should not be an over-formalized or elaborate task. Whilst it is self-evident that any employer will want a new employee to be trained for the job and to settle into the working environment, it is too readily assumed that all this will occur naturally and automatically. In part this is because the doctors themselves often had to find their feet in a variety of jobs without any direct assistance, and it is thus assumed that others will 'sink or swim' in much the same way. In fact it is in the GPs' own interests as the employer to ensure that the new recruit 'swims' as quickly and effectively as possible, and does not 'sink' because her training has been neglected.

Continuing education

Training does not, of course, end when induction is completed. The increasing demands on general practice today means that it is essential for practice staff to be encouraged to update and develop their skills and knowledge. There are a wide range of training and continuity education courses available for practice staff. The Association of Medical Secretaries, Practice Administrators and Receptionists (AMSPAR), runs many courses for practice staff. Advice can be obtained from this body at: Tavistock House (North), Tavistock Square, London WC1H 9LN. The Association of Health Centre and Practice Administrations (AHCPA) is also active in this and may be contacted at The Royal College of General Practitioners, 14 Princes Gate, Hyde Park, London SW7 1PU. Radcliffe Medical Press, 15 Kings Meadow, Ferry Hinksey Road, Oxford OX2 0DP runs Practice Receptionist Programme, Practice Manager Development, Practice Computer Training, Financial Management in Practice and Practice Nurse Programme.

Training is not however simply a matter of attending and acquiring formal qualifications. Informal practice meetings can make an important contribution to staff education, particularly if care is taken to ensure that the subject matter relates to the work of the practice team. These meetings can be particularly beneficial if they are sufficiently informal to encourage staff to contribute to the discussion.

4 The Nature of Management and Administration

Introduction

GENERAL practice managers are unique. The majority of managers—there were over 2½ million of them in 1988—work in a specific function within a large organization, either in the private or the public sector. They may be working in departments of finance, personnel, research and development, production, marketing and distribution, sales or after-sales service. They will be responsible for one particular aspect of their firm's work. For example, an individual personnel manager may be responsible for the pay and conditions of non-manual staff. Here, they will be directly responsible to a more senior manager, the departmental head, and through him to more senior managers (there are characteristically seven levels of managers in a large organization, although there may be as many as 12). In addition, the individual manager may have a 'dotted line' relationship with yet another senior manager. For example, the plant personnel manager is responsible on a day-to-day basis to the plant director, and to the senior personnel director at head office for overall policy.

The general practice manager works in a quite different setting. She is part of a large public sector organization, the National Health Service, which is the largest employer in Europe. However, she will work in a relatively small organization, with perhaps up to ten staff. The number of practices with five or more partners is increasing, and such practices may have as many as 40 staff in total, but such large practices are not the most common. It is estimated that only 10 000 of Britain's 32 000 GPs work in practices with four or more partners. Unlike most managers, the practice manager will have a much wider range of responsibilities: for people, for money, for office procedures, for relations with patients, for relations with other medical agencies, and for dealing with the general public. She will not be helped, and protected, by a large staff of assistants. She may have clearly defined responsibilities, set out in a detailed job description, but more likely she will not. She may have a managing partner to report to, but it is more likely that she will be equally responsible to all partners, all of whom have other major interests and responsibilities. She may have a number of assistants who handle a limited range of management responsibilities, for example finance, but again it is more likely that she will not.

The practice manager is therefore a special kind of manager, working in a small unit, with wide responsibilities and in direct contact with the general public. Her work is especially challenging, and especially visible.

The practice manager is special, but she remains a manager, with normal management responsibilities and tasks. The essence of management lies in establishing objectives, translating objectives into roles, tasks and procedures, establishing priorities, and ensuring that the objectives are achieved. This involves dealing with a wide range of people and issues, and establishing priorities between them. It involves ensuring that decisions are not ignored, or changed without thought the following month. Inside the practice the practice manager, like all managers, has to look upwards to the partners, sideways to the other practice managers and downwards to other employees of the practice. She also has to look outside the organization, to patients, to other parts of the Health Service, and to the surrounding community.

The rest of this chapter explains these general matters more fully and covers seven elements.

1 Establishing objectives.
2 Defining roles, tasks and procedures.
3 Establishirg priorities.
4 Securing and allocating resources.
5 Securing compliance.
6 Monitoring performance.
7 Watching the outside world.

Establishing objectives

The specific objectives of practices may vary, and there may be differences between partners in the same practice. However, it is important that the practice should have objectives discussed and if possible agreed among the partners. This is especially important if the practice is considering the selection of a new partner, or is engaged in continuing education. Among the questions which need to be asked are: Who should define the objectives? What are the objectives and how precisely should they be defined? How often should they be reviewed? How important is it to be able to measure performance against the objectives? Should the objectives be stated in financial terms? What other measurements are appropriate?

Who should define the objectives? There is a difference between the aims of a practice and the objectives of a practice, although the two words are often used to mean the same thing. The aims of the practice may be very general to promote good health and prevent disease whenever possible. The partners are directly responsible for establishing such overall aims for the practice just as the Board of Directors is responsible for establishing the aims of a public corporation. It is not the responsibility of the practice manager to say what the aims should be, although she might have to ensure that some explicit aims exist, such as that tetanus immunization should be offered to all patients every ten years, and are discussed from time to time. But it is the responsibility of the practice manager to translate overall aims into more specific objectives, and to secure agreement from the partners that the objectives are a satisfactory method for meeting the practice's aims.

Corporation directors may define the aims of the corporation as being 'to provide technological leadership for the industry' (first of the pack) or to be at the forefront in terms of 'quality of service' (as the Lex company, which operates in leasing, has done). This is translated into the objective of being able to respond to all requests for service within a given time period. Medical practices are not public corporations, concerned with profits and market share, but they require an idea of how to translate good health care into practical terms, and to assess whether they are being successful or not. The practical measure of good health care might be reviewing all diabetic patients at agreed intervals, or limiting the delays between patients telephoning for an appointment and seeing the doctor. If possible, the objectives should be measureable by making use of information which the practice would require for other reasons, rather than establishing special requirements.

Once established, the aims of the practice should only be reviewed at long intervals. However, the objectives might be appropriately reviewed on a bi-annual basis, depending upon the frequency of changes in the practice's environment. Reviewing the objectives too frequently can be wasteful, especially if little has changed for the practice.

Business organizations typically establish a target rate of return on assets, and may establish a target market share. Practice managers will find it difficult to follow established business practice, since they are not operating in a market. However, it may be helpful to establish financial targets. If targets are established they should not be established solely in terms of costs, but in terms of returns on assets; otherwise there is the danger of being totally preoccupied with reductions in costs rather than the realization of benefits. For example, the purchase of a new ECG machine might be assessed by the use to which it is put.

Defining roles, tasks and procedures

The precise distribution of work within the practice will depend upon several factors, especially the size of the practice, the number and qualifications of the staff, the physical arrangements of the surgery, waiting room, reception area and office, and many other things. The larger the practice, and the larger the staff, the greater the importance of having clearly defined roles, tasks and procedures. However, as practices are very busy, and even practices with a few partners may have large numbers of part-time staff, it is important for matters to be defined clearly. It is especially important for the roles, tasks and procedures to be documented as there is likely to be significant turnover of staff, perhaps including turnover in practice managers.

There are three general questions.

Who is to define roles, tasks and procedures?
How closely should they be defined?
What considerations need to be taken into account when establishing the structure?

It is the practice manager's job to define the roles, tasks and procedures within the practice, except where there are clear medical issues involved. The practice manager should be familiar with the requirements of good practice management, which involves a knowledge of general office practice as well as specific features of general practice. The partners should be informed and consulted, but there is no reason to expect that GPs should be experts in management (any more than practice managers need medical qualifications). It may be helpful in group practices if one of the partners fulfils the function of the managing partner in an accountancy practice, but this role is not necessarily one which must be filled by the senior partner. It might also be helpful if one partner takes on, say, financial aspects, another education and so on but defined lines of communication should exist to avoid confusion.

Some business organizations are structured like a machine, with everything clearly defined; other business organizations operate on more 'organic' principles, with members of staff assuming a wide range of responsibilities, without clear definition. The first type of system works best when it is possible to predict what will happen perhaps because the firm is making a simple product for a known market (like bread); the second type of organization works best when circumstances are frequently changing, perhaps because of changes in technology or because the market is unpredictable (like high fashion clothing). Patients' symptoms are varied, and the job of the GP is not programmed. However, the organization of the practice can be programmed, as patients are dealt with in standard portions of time. The roles and tasks of members of staff, and the procedures to be followed, can therefore be relatively programmed and worked out on a clearly defined basis. This is particularly necessary where staff are relatively inexperienced or are working on a part-time basis and do not have the opportunity to familiarize themselves fully with the procedures followed in the surgery. There are good legal reasons as well why care protocols should be explicit for staff.

The interests of the employee as well as the interests of the partners and the patients should be taken into account when establishing patterns of work. This is especially important where the practice manager needs employees to adopt a flexible attitude towards their work, for example over standing in for other staff who are off sick or with family difficulties and when it is difficult to predict when work in an evening will end. If staff interests are ignored it is difficult to expect them to adopt a flexible attitude. The final responsibility rests with the practice manager, but she should take a wide range of interests into account and motivation becomes very important.

In many organizations the general public is invisible, or only dealt with by a small number of employees. However, in general practice the public, as patients, is centrally involved, and the practice employees are in the public eye at a time when the patient has a high level of anxiety. It is therefore necessary to pay attention to 'patient management' as well as to 'staff management' when deciding on the allocation of roles and tasks; front office as well as back office skills are required. This makes a flexible approach even more necessary.

Establishing priorities

Practice managers will always find themselves with too much to do and too little time to do it. Their staff will find the same problem. It is the practice manager's job to establish priorities, both for herself and for other members of staff. The manager's job falls into four broad types of activity; (a) report preparation; (b) internal communication; (c) external communication; and (d) meetings. The manager's work is fragmented, and only a relatively small amount of time is spent thinking or planning, or on the preparation of reports, even in large organizations. This is likely to be even more true in small organizations. However, it is important for the practice manager to avoid spending all the time dealing with yesterday's crisis, and working in a fragmented way. Spending time establishing priorities should reduce the amount of time which has to be spent in responding to yesterday's crisis. The practice manager will also need to balance pressures coming from different quarters—from doctors, other staff, patients, administrators, officials and doctors in other medical institutions. The highest immediate priority might not always be the priority established by the partners.

The specific priorities of the practice manager will vary between practices. Some practices will have a different range of issues to deal with than others, perhaps because of the clinical facilities available in the particular catchment area in which the practice is located. The establishment of medical priorities is the responsibility of the practice partners. However, the medical priorities chosen all have financial and organizational consequences and it is the job of the practice manager to establish what these are and to make them clear to the partners. There is usually a range of activities necessary for supporting the medical activities of the practice which will be primarily the responsibility of the practice manager and she is directly responsible for establishing priorities in this area.

In business organizations it is possible to establish priorities on the basis of financial criteria such as reductions in the costs of production or contributions to an increase in sales. There are some equivalents in medical practices. The costs of running the practice (staff, equipment, property costs) can be assessed and compared with the costs of other practices. It is possible to assess the effectiveness of the practice in ensuring that fees and reimbursements from the FHSA are maximized. It is, of course, also possible to assess the performance of the practice with private patients in directly economic terms.

It is particularly important to have clearly established priorities when recruiting new staff, or when investing in new equipment. When appointing new staff there is an obvious practice of simply replacing the person who has left. However, vacancies provide an opportunity to assess the overall position of the practice, and to consider whether the staffing requirements have changed since the last appointment was made. Could the work of existing staff be rearranged, either to reduce the time taken by different tasks, or to broaden the experience of existing staff? This may be a good way of making the work more interesting, as well as making it easier to cover for other staff during absences. If new staff are appointed, it might be desirable to appoint a different type of person from the person who left, perhaps to change the age distribution of staff or to introduce new skills.

The same policy of reconsidering the total picture should be adopted when buying major new pieces of equipment. In particular, the increased sophistication and reduced cost of computers has made it possible to record and store information in more efficient ways than in the past. It is possible to combine functions which had previously to be done by different people. Computerizing the practice office may be inappropriate, because it is too expensive, or because it requires too highly skilled staff, or because the working conditions in the office are too confusing for the staff to cope with the complex equipment. However, it may be that substantial improvements in efficiency are possible and as practices become more involved in the care of groups of patients, hypertensives, diabetics, asthmatics, the elderly, immunization or paediatric surveillance for example, it may become essential. The important point is not to establish an electronic office in inappropriate circumstances, but to ensure that equipment purchases are looked at in the overall context of practice requirements, for the present and the future, and not undertaken on a simple replacement basis. If the practice manager does not consider such issues, no-one else is likely to.

Hiring new staff and buying new equipment are activities common to many types of managers. But the practice manager has the difficult task of ensuring that changes which improve business efficiency do not damage patient satisfaction. The practice manager has to establish priorities where the overall objectives may not be clear-cut. In particular, medical and financial requirements have to be reconciled. It is therefore more important for the practice manager than for anyone else that the objectives of the practice should be clear, for without such guidance her job becomes impossible.

The basis for establishing priorities in business organizations is usually provided by the budget. The budget is conventionally divided into capital and operating expenditures. The practice manager has to establish priorities within the framework of the practice budget.

Securing and allocating resources

The practice manager is responsible for the preparation of the annual budget and for securing fees and reimbursements from the FHSA. The practice manager should have an annual budget, and a longer term planning horizon for major expenditures, say three years. It is impossible to consider major investments, for example in computerization, unless a time scale longer than 12 months is taken into account. In addition, the practice manager is responsible for the day-to-day control of the expenditure, although not necessarily involved in the recording or authorization of specific expenditures and receipts.

In business organizations the budget has two functions. First, it acts as a financial tool, involving estimates of future expenditures, both capital and operating, and future income. This is obviously necessary to ensure that the business does not run into financial difficulties, and is the major means of providing guidance for individual managers. Secondly, as a planning tool, as a way of representing the priorities of the business.

The practice budget is, however, different from the budget of a business organization. In business organizations the budget is related to anticipated income from the sale of the firm's products or services. The practice's level of income is determined largely by the level of fees and allowances provided by the NHS, apart from any income from private patients. The 'price' is determined by the buyer, not the provider of the service. This makes it more difficult for the practice manager to predict future income, particularly over a period longer than 12 months. However, the preparation of a financial plan, including an annual budget, remains essential.

The first major resource required by the practice manager is money. The practice manager is also responsible for the provision of physical facilities: support facilities, including reception facilities, and office facilities. These are the second resource available. The precise equipment required will vary from practice to practice, according to the size of the partnership, the length of the patient list, the frequency of patient visits to the surgery, the number and competence of staff, and other factors. The practice manager's concern is with 'fitness for purpose'. Consideration needs to be given to the costs of service and maintenance as well as to the costs of the initial purchase. Again, it is important to consider the overall requirements of the practice.

The third major resource is staff time, both the practice manager's own and that of other members of staff. The preparation of an annual and a weekly schedule is again the responsibility of the practice manager; time management is a significant management responsibility, frequently taught on management programmes. The preparation of an annual calendar should give the practice manager the opportunity to review the workings of the practice with the partners. The review should cover the work of the practice manager herself, as well as the work of other members of staff. The practice manager will also need a weekly timetable. The details of the weekly timetable may change throughout the year, but again should be agreed with the partner who acts as 'managing partner' for the practice.

The timetable of clinical staff, doctors, employed practice nurses and attached staff who may use practice premises at times (such as health visitors, district nurses, a speech therapist, clinical psychologist, etc.) dictate the work-load coming through. The need to plan support staff for these activities as well as the other office or administrative activities is referred to in the paragraphs below.

The weekly timetable should include provision for a regular partner meeting, to cover the workings of the practice. The meetings may be informal, but records should be kept by the practice manager to ensure that decisions are carried forward.

The allocation of resources should be closely tied to the priorities of the practice. However, it is important to remember that issues may be of considerable importance, even if they are never the top priority; office support facilities may never be the top of the list, but provide a necessary basis for the effectiveness of the overall practice. Resources need to be provided for the infrastructure of the practice, even if it is difficult to justify the cost of the infrastructure in conventional financial or indeed in medical terms.

Securing compliance

Securing compliance refers to the process of ensuring that the practice manager's wishes are carried out by other staff. It is not enough to 'make decisions' or to say 'do this' and to assume that your wishes will be carried out. In large industrial organizations securing compliance is a major problem, involving complex systems of supervision. Securing compliance is easier in small organizations, like medical practices. The practice manager can use her own personality and knowledge of individuals to build up loyalty and willingness to co-operate amongst the staff—the practice manager is not a remote name. The practice manager should be able to treat the staff as individuals. However, compliance cannot be taken for granted even in small organizations; it has to be sought and kept actively. This may be more difficult in general practice than in other small organizations because of the wide variety of staff including many part-time staff, with very different backgrounds and interests—medical, nursing, secretarial, as well as cleaning and repair staff. The pressure of large numbers of patients in the surgery is a further source of tension, making it important for the practice manager to be sensitive to the individual needs of the staff. A common problem is that decisions made at practice meetings are not followed through so the practice manager has to secure 'compliance' amongst doctors with their own decisions. How is this achieved?

Staff work for different reasons, and respond to different approaches. The main reason for complying with the wishes of the practice manager is custom and practice: it is expected. However, practices can become inefficient if practice managers become careless and begin to take compliance for granted. Compliance can become only nominal and provide a poor basis for an effective practice. Staff who work in general practice may have different approaches to work from staff who work in other organizations, and therefore accept orders for different reasons. In particular, the image of a caring profession will be important to many members of staff, and the approach adopted by the practice manager should reflect that approach. This is important for administrative as well as for medical and nursing staff. Such administrative staff, secretaries, receptionists and clerks, may be especially important, particularly in London and the south of England, because here they could obtain jobs in quite different lines of work—perhaps less interesting, but also less stressful and more remunerative. Even whilst adopting a financially realistic approach, the practice manager should not forget this caring orientation.

Different staff supervisors have different styles, some more authoritarian than others. The supervisory style should reflect the personality of the practice manager, the orientations of the staff, and the particular working environment of general practice. The need to ensure calm working relationships when working under pressure means that a very authoritarian approach is likely to lead to major difficulties, and especially to high levels of staff turnover; it is very wasteful for the practice to lose staff, since it takes time to learn the particular ways of operating of different practices.

The details of staff management are discussed in Chapter 6. Here the concern is simply to stress the importance of paying attention to the need to ensure compliance, and to secure that compliance actively.

Monitoring performance

The practice manager needs to ensure that the practice is working both effectively and efficiently. Effectively means achieving the overall objectives of the practice, efficiently means achieving this at minimum cost. This involves monitoring the performance of the practice as a whole, and of individual members of staff. This can only be done if the objectives of the practice are clear, priorities established and roles and tasks clearly defined.

The establishment of the overall aims of the practice is the responsibility of the partners. The partners should also be responsible for agreeing to the measures of performance established to monitor the overall performance of the practice. This is very similar to the audit of clinical activities that clinical staff are involved with. Just as they have to measure what they do to see if it can be done better so do administrative staff and very frequently the two activities are intertwined. The practice manager may suggest possible measures, or indicate why some possible measures are inappropriate, perhaps because it would be difficult to keep information in the form required. The practice manager should ensure that information is available to the partners in a form which enables them to see how the practice is doing, and in a form which they can readily understand. In monitoring performance, comparable figures from a previous year, or from a comparable practice if available, should be provided. Partners do not wish to be overburdened with information, but the provision of basic information quarterly, with the possibility of having it available monthly, is one possible approach.

The practice manager is responsible for monitoring the performance of individual members of staff. She should avoid too heavy an emphasis upon formal monitoring of performance, because staff then begin to work to the performance criteria rather than to the requirements of the job, ignoring important parts of the job which may happen not to be measured. Formal monitoring should also be less necessary in a small organization than in a large organization, because the manager in a small organization has the possibility of directly observing the work of individual members of staff. However, increasing government concern with the costs of general practice may lead to the establishment of formal criteria of assessment for staff, as a condition for the reimbursement of costs, even if the assessment is unnecessary in terms of the practical operation of the practice. In the long run formal schemes of job evaluation may be established, which would involve assessments of the levels of skill and experience required, as well as the actual difficulty of the job. In the short run, practice managers should discuss systematically the performance of individual members of staff with the staff concerned at least once a year. This discussion should review the individual's work throughout the year, and should be separate from any discussion of salary, promotion or regrading.

The practice is a business, as well as a public service. The performance of the practice as a business will therefore have to be monitored. Such monitoring should focus on the performance of the practice against the budget. Comparisons of performance against budget may be made monthly or quarterly in business organizations; a similar frequency might be appropriate for a large practice.

Watching the outside world

The individual practice is a small part of a large organization. Its fortunes are very directly dependent upon its links with the outside world; hospitals, NHS administrative agencies, public health authorities, local authorities, other medical practitioners, as well as patients; the full range of relevant institutions is touched upon in later chapters. The doctors have a wide range of links with the medical world but it is also the practice manager's job to maintain contacts with the outside world, especially the non-medical world, and to be informed about changes which affect the practice. She must know what changes are being made by the DHA, for example alterations of clinic times, changed access to diagnostic facilities, appointments of new consultants and published lists of waiting times. She must be aware of changes initiated by the FHSA and think how every alteration in the terms and conditions of service might influence practice activity now and in the longer term. She must also watch the journals that come in to the practice for many of these provide information about practice activity elsewhere. Finally, she must be aware of changes in the local community around the practice. There is a major danger that the practice manager will be too inward looking, at a time when major threats to the practice are likely to come from outside.

The practice manager must obviously be aware of changes in the NHS which are likely to affect the practice. Changes in the financial arrangements governing the practice will have a direct impact upon the job of the practice manager. Closer monitoring of the financial performance will have a direct impact upon the practice manager, requiring the provision of more financial information than has been required in the past. Full budgetary responsibility for the individual practice would involve a very substantial increase in the responsibilities of the practice manager. Changes in the NHS will require the attention of the partners in the practice; but it will be the responsibility of the practice manager to ensure that up-to-date, accurate and full information is available to the partnership.

Other changes in the outside world will have a major impact upon the practice. Some of the changes will affect the 'patient mix' and therefore the likely pattern of surgery visits, for example if there is a major change in the age or social composition of the population in the area covered by the practice. New housing developments, or even simply changes in the price of houses in the district, may have significant implications for the practice. Many such changes will be known to the partners: but it is the practice manager's specific responsibility to be informed. Doctors are over-burdened with too much information.

To summarize, management is a process of decision making, involving seven elements.

1 Establishing objectives.
2 Defining roles, tasks and procedures.
3 Establishing priorities.
4 Securing and allocating resources.
5 Securing compliance.
6 Monitoring performance.
7 Watching the environment.

These basic management processes are the same, whether the manager is working in a large industrial organization or in a medical practice. Some of the elements require almost continuous awareness, especially monitoring performance and watching the environment. Some involve only occasional attention, establishing objectives and defining roles, tasks and procedures. However, each element requires attention at least annually.

Administration

Management is a decision-making activity, involving the choice between alternatives. Once decisions have been made, carrying them through involves administration. Administration is the establishment of rules and procedures, and applying those rules and procedures in particular cases. For example, specifying how repeat prescriptions should be dealt with, after the criteria have been laid down, and seeing that repeat prescriptions are made for individual patients in accordance with the rules specified.

Establishing rules and procedures and enforcing them may be bureaucratic, and bureaucracy is unpopular, especially with patients. Practice managers are therefore faced with the problem of balancing the requirements of administrative efficiency against the pressure to treat patients as individual, special cases. Too little flexibility is inhumane, too much flexibility leads to favouritism and difficulties in overall patient handling. It is necessary to judge when a patient's claim for priority attention is justified or not. Different practices will have different procedures and ways of administering the procedures, influenced by the partners and, especially, by the practice manager. Experience in non-medical organizations suggests five general comments.

Firstly, rules and procedures can only be developed when things happen regularly; it is impossible to develop rules for the unexpected, and a waste of time to develop rules for things which happen very infrequently. When establishing procedures it is necessary to consider how predictable an event is, and how often it occurs. The medical support, office and reception area activities of general practice involve large numbers of predictable and frequent events, and it is therefore desirable, and economical in time, to develop clear and relatively extensive formal procedures.

Secondly, the impact on staff of methods of administration needs to be considered. The development of rigid rules and procedures limits the scope for the exercise of initiative and discretion by practice staff. If they are always required to do exactly what the rule book tells them to do they are less likely to be willing, or able, to assume direct responsibility, even in an emergency, than if they are encouraged to make their own decisions. However, practice staff are dealing with patients under stress, and it may be helpful to staff to have the rule book to rely upon when under pressure from patients, to 'know where they stand'. It is much easier, and more acceptable to say that 'the rules don't allow it' than it is to say 'I don't allow it'. Examples will include the rules about making appointments, responding to requests for home visits, patients speaking to doctors on the telephone, handling emergencies and so on. Moreover, there is a major need for continuity when large numbers of part-time staff are employed; this requires carefully worked out and clear procedures which can be relatively quickly learned. The chances of mistakes occurring through lack of knowledge of the practice are high, especially when large numbers of part-time staff are employed together.

Thirdly, the impact of administration on patients needs to be considered. Patients have conflicting wishes; the wish to be treated as special, as an individual, and the wish to be treated the same as everybody else, fairly. The first wish requires leaving a wide range of discretion to individual members of staff (for example on how urgently to make an appointment). The second wish involves specifying the rules fully (for example saying that priority appointments may only be made under specified circumstances).

Discretion must be given to staff to deal with emergencies, and to decide when an emergency is a real emergency. On the other hand, it is easier for a patient to complain that he or she was discriminated against and treated unfairly when there are no rules which state how a patient should be treated; the rules provide the criteria for judging whether the patient was treated fairly or not.

Fourthly, the impact of methods of administration upon the practice itself, and especially the ability to assess how efficiently the practice is working, needs to be considered. If procedures are unclear it is difficult to know whether 'best practice' is being followed or not, and if staff time is being used efficiently. This links in with the importance of monitoring performance.

Finally, formal procedures will be increasingly important as the NHS concerns itself more with 'good management' and 'value for money'. Practices will need to demonstrate to outsiders that they are providing value for money. It is easier to demonstrate 'value for money' if there are clear administrative procedures than if wide areas are left to individual discretion. Practices which leave large areas of discretion to individual members of staff, and fail to provide adequate training, will be especially likely to be criticized. It is also the best protection against charges from outside that mistakes have been made and care not provided of an adequate standard.

The development of information technology is having a direct impact upon practice administration. Repeat prescribing is now computerized in nearly 50% of all practices. Some form of clinical record-keeping is computerized in 30% and systems for managing appointment systems and financial systems are being introduced. These do not often make less work and they usually make more but they do improve the quality of what is done and make it possible to obtain data about what is going on within the practice for audit purposes. Newer and more sophisticated systems will be required as the role of general practice continues to expand and as links are developed between data held by DHAs, FHSAs and the practice itself. Information on performance will be required both for good practice and in order to demonstrate good practice.

Conclusion

The general practice is a small organization, working within the framework of a very large organization. This is the type of pattern which many large business organizations are trying to establish as the most efficient form of organization 'small within large'. This presents the practice manager with many opportunities, as well as difficulties. This concluding section outlines the opportunities and difficulties which face the practice manager compared with the manager in a large industrial organization.

The practice manager is the member of a small team. She is able to know the other members of the team as individuals, and to build up close working relations with them. This makes it easier to develop commitment to the practice. With a small team it is possible to develop a flexible approach to work, with members of the practice encouraged to learn about the whole range of practice activities. Small size means that there is no need to waste time passing information up a chain of command, and waiting perhaps for months for decisions. Personal relationships, and personal feelings, are important. At the same time, the practice has access to the resources of a very large organization, the NHS. This is a source of expertise, advice and assistance, as well as finance.

Although the practice is small, it is not simple. Although there are only a small number of staff, they have very different skills, and they are not interchangeable. There are therefore limits to the job flexibility which is possible. Moreover, the pressures under which doctors work means that it is not always possible to secure their attention for practice management problems, and to obtain necessary decisions. Finally, the NHS imposes many requirements upon practices, not all of which are helpful to the practice itself, as well as providing resources.

The practice manager is a 'negotiator' between the different groups involved in the practice—the partners, the staff, the patients, the NHS. Each has to be satisfied if the practice is to work effectively. The partners are the major 'stakeholders' and if they are not satisfied the practice manager is not likely to remain in the practice for very long. But the other stakeholders need to be satisfied also in the long run if the practice is to survive. The practice manager therefore needs to consider the interests of all stakeholders and to consider how to reconcile their often conflicting interests.

This task of negotiation is similar to that of managers in other organizations. However, there are five features which make the task of the practice manager different from the task of other managers.

Firstly, she is responsible for a wide range of tasks, which would be divided between different departments in a larger organization—finance, personnel, purchasing, office management, relations with the public. This makes the job in some ways easier, since she does not have to consult with a wide range of other managers. But it also makes it more demanding, since she is responsible for such a variety of relationships.

Secondly, she is responsible for a wide range of staff—nursing, secretarial, cleaning and maintenance. This again requires awareness of a wide range of issues; different grades of staff have different skills, interests, and pay scales. If large numbers of part-time staff are employed there is the additional problem of arranging work schedules. Staff management is especially important because of the importance of staff sensitivity to patient needs.

Thirdly, she will be involved in dealing with the general public, at a time when they are experiencing personal stress. This is likely to lead to tension in the reception area, especially if the doctors are unable to keep to the appointments timetable. The practice manager will be working 'in public', and may be called upon to handle tensions between her staff and members of the public.

Fourthly, the practice manager has little control over the major factors which determine the income of the practice. The business manager is able to determine the price of his product according to the costs of the production, the prices charged by competitors, and generally by 'what the market will bear'. The practice manager is tied to a scale of fees and reimbursements determined by the FHSA, and in commercial terms is operating with one hand tied behind her back. She is able to influence the expenditures of the practice, but not to have an equivalent influence on the income.

Finally, the practice manager has little influence over the institutional context in which the practice operates. The context is provided by the NHS, and the NHS operates within a complex legislative framework. The practice manager has to be aware of the ways in which the NHS affects the practice, but has little opportunity to influence the wider organization. There is little opportunity for the practice manager to look for new markets!

The practice manager is, then, a special kind of manager. She is required to perform the same management tasks as other managers but she is operating in a unique environment, with its own constraints and opportunities. The remainder of this book provides advice on how to manage in these special circumstances.

5   The Role of the Practice Manager

WE are concerned in this chapter with the interface between the practice manager and the other staff in the practice. The practice manager lies at the very centre of the practice, interfacing with all the other people and organizations who form the primary health care team. The model (Fig. 5.1) illustrates this central role. The practice manager has the responsibility for co-ordinating the way in which primary care is delivered in the practice.

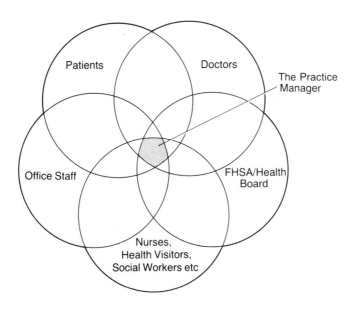

Figure 5.1   Interface between staff, patients and the doctor.

Each territory interfaces with all the others. For which interface should the manager be the medium? For some there would be little dispute; the doctor might prefer that the manager performs all the interactions with the FHSA, the district nurse may see little role for the manager in her consultations with the doctor. Some situations are straightforward and will not cause ill-feeling. Others are more difficult; a doctor may feel that he should tick off a receptionist who is not doing her job properly. Where does this leave the practice manager who has the responsibility for dealing with the staff? This and many other interactions, where the practice manager feels that it is her place in the practice to co-ordinate, will cause problems.

We must consider just what the place of the practice manager is. The task has changed dramatically in the last year, the speed of change having been accelerated by the 1990 GP Contract. The old style of practice administrator still remains of course, and for many administration will continue to be the bulk of the job. However for others, and particularly in larger practices, the expanded role of practice management will require a fresh approach to the division of work. The task of deciding how roles within the practice are shared out is not easy. It is however, made simpler by the use of a number of tools, common to management practice everywhere. They are:

- Meetings.
- Rotas.
- Job descriptions.
- Training and appraisal.
- Partnership agreements.

The interface with the doctor

The doctor–manager interface is often considered to be the most trying. The problem stems from the role of the doctor as owner of the business and one who draws his income from it. In delegating work to the manager the doctor takes a financial gamble. This is, of course, more true now that FHSAs have staff budgets. Furthermore, the doctor has an authority problem, 'can I trust this person to deal with my affairs?'. The practice manager will need to bear in mind the delicate ego that underlies these dilemmas.

In the interface between doctors and the manager, her sphere of influence should include all those areas that may impinge on the patients or on the staff.

- Length of surgeries.
- Time of surgeries.
- Doctors' holidays.

- Partnership disputes.
- Sick doctors.
- Complaints against doctors.

These are all delicate matters. No wonder then that this area of influence is hotly contested!

A number of tools exist to assist the manager in dealing with the difficult and disputed areas of interest. Without them the practice manager finds herself handicapped by not knowing the right way to approach a problem. The tools are not unfamiliar ones.

- Partnership agreements.
- Practice meetings.
- Rotas.

Partnership agreements

Doctors who choose to practice in partnerships do so for a number of reasons. Firstly, for sociability – professional life in isolation is onerous. Secondly, for convenience – a principal in practice delivers 24-hour care for 365 days a year. Being in a partnership means sharing night duty, afternoons off and study leave, all much more difficult for the single-handed practitioner. Thirdly, to aid the division of labour – the partnership can have a variety of sub-specialists whose skills vary but complement each other.

Where there are benefits, there are usually costs and a price to be paid. The cost is loss of autonomy. Partnerships mean sharing – sharing work, decision-making and money. When one partner does more, another does less. In a dispute about policy, share of profits or share of work the partner who does not 'win the day' feels reduced by the decision. He has, by taking on the responsibility of the partnership, given up his own autonomy for that of the joint autonomy. He cannot act for himself to the exclusion of the others. Partnership is a marriage.

In order to make partnerships fair, so that partners feel less aggrieved by the work of the partnership, many practices have a written and formal agreement between the doctors involved. This is not universal. Many doctors take the view that, being friends and professionals, and sharing the same values, such an agreement is not necessary. They are often right, but partnership disputes do arise, even in the happiest of practices. Some examples of scenarios follow.

1 A partner obtains sessional work in a factory as industrial medical officer. Because the work is over lunchtime and does not intrude on practice time, he elects to keep the income to himself and not to share it in the partnership. The others feel aggrieved. Who is right?

2   A partner, by virtue of a slipped disc, takes prolonged sick leave. Not having any sickness or locum insurance, the burden of the work falls on the other partners. It is unclear when he will return. What action can be taken?

3   A partner appears to take two weeks leave more than the others. Should they take more, or he less?

All these, and many other worse scenarios should fall within the jurisdiction of a Deed of Partnership which should clearly set out the agreed procedure. The following areas are routinely included in such agreements, which are usually drawn up by a solicitor under the direction of the partners. All partners are then signatories to the agreement which legally binds them. Many practices find that the existence of such an agreement prevents potentially damaging disputes arising, since the rules are already clear and not subject to debate.

What then, should be included in the Deed of Partnership? Statements should be made about all the following:

1   The names of the partners signatory to the agreement.

2   The site at which they practice.

3   The ownership of the premises and the fixtures, fittings and drugs at that premises.

4   A statement about provision of cars; do they belong to the practice or are they the private property of the doctors? Does the practice pay for the maintenance and running of the cars, or do the doctors do so as private individuals?

5   What items shall be expenses of the partnership? Examples might be rent and rates, loan repayments, stationery, drugs, accountancy, practice telephone bills. Will the partnership pay for partners private telephone bills?

6   Where does the partnership bank? What monies should go into that account? Will monies earned outside of the partners' list be part of the partnership income or will it be kept by that partner?

7   Who will keep the practice accounts?

8   What share of the profits of the practice will be due to each partner? It is unusual for new and junior doctors to receive the same share as senior partners. A more usual arrangement is for the junior partner to gradually increase his share of the profits over two or three years until he becomes a full or 'parity' partner.

9   How much holiday can each partner take each year? How much study leave may he take?

10 How long will the practice elect to bear the burden of a doctor absent through sickness? Must each doctor insure against such sickness and arrange to pay locum fees while away?

11   What happens if a doctor becomes mentally ill (for example, nervous breakdown) such that his patients are at risk? Does the partnership have the right to dissolve the partnership and reconstitute it without him?
12   What notice of retirement is needed?
13   In the case of partnership disputes without apparent solution who can be appointed arbitrator?

Partnership agreements never cover all eventualities. They are a measure of the commitment of each partner to the others. Their existence is a bond between the partners; they should not be used as a stick with which to beat each other. It is often said that once a partnership has to consult its agreement the partnership is finished. This need not be the case; partnerships, like marriages and friendships, go through good and bad patches. The presence of the agreement ensures that in a bad patch the partners know what action to take to avoid a damaging split. Of course partnerships do dissolve even if they have apparently watertight agreements. Human nature dictates that sometimes people just cannot agree. The merit of the legally binding agreement is that it ensures an equitable solution even if the worst does come to the worst.

The importance of the partnership agreement to the practice manager lies, then, in its existence. The detail included in it need not be known to her; it is after all an agreement between the doctors. Its value for her is as a tool to be used when necessary, to be drawn attention to when it seems to be called for. In a practice without one she should be advocating it and providing guidelines for those areas where it seems to be needed most. This is part of her pro-active role; not waiting for an accident to happen, but anticipating it and pre-empting it by advising on standard practice. This is good management.

Good practices do not wait for problems to occur, fall out over the solutions and consult the partnership agreement for the quickest way to split the profits and run. They predict problems, act pro-actively and review their actions in the light of experience. How do they set about doing so?

Practice meetings

The practice meeting is the embodiment of our model of the practice. Here the practice meets to discuss the interfaces between the patients, doctors and the staff. The practice meeting is a wonderful opportunity to meet, discuss and to make decisions. It may not fulfil any of these functions if the organization behind it fails. About any group of regular meetings the following questions need to be addressed.

1   frequency;
2   place;

3　time;
4　who is invited;
5　agenda;
6　chairman.

Ad hoc meetings in the corridor between two or more members of a practice are barely adequate. They lead to ill feeling amongst those not privy to the 'decision' and the decision may be useless because the important people have not been consulted.

Frequency, place and time

Practice meetings must occur at the time when the most, and preferably all, of the parties concerned can be present. This sounds like common sense, it sounds obvious and straightforward but it is neither. Nobody wants to trail back into the practice in the evening but not everybody comes if the meeting is at lunchtime. Of course there are sensible compromises but compromise may not be a virtue attached to your practice. Frequency is best judged by the size of the agenda; if there is too much to discuss without curtailing some agenda items the meetings need to be more frequent.

Agenda

Meetings without an agenda are doomed to failure. An agenda means that the parties present have had time to consider their views on an item, rather than making 'off the cuff' prejudicial judgments. An agenda says, 'These items will be discussed today. If you have a veiw you wish to express this is the time to do it.' It also says, 'only these items will be discussed today; any others will have to wait until next week.' 'Any other business' is not the time to start debating the merits or otherwise of the new diabetic clinic. A good agenda list should include the names of those who asked for a topic to be included. There are few more wearying sights than a chairman asking, 'Who wants to speak on this . . . . ?' The agenda should be available and delivered two days before the meeting.

Chairman

The job of the chairman is to keep the meeting to the agenda, to make sure that it is cleared (finished), to ensure that everyone who wants to speak does so and that those who wish to speak all the time do not. Chairmen may be permanent (often custom and practice makes this the senior partner) or rotating. There is a good case for practice managers chairing meetings. The role of chairman strictly implies no seniority whatsoever, since his or her task is simply to keep the meeting to order. Anything else is an abuse of authority.

Minutes must be taken; subjectivity and memory are the enemies of good management. Objectivity is the key. If decisions are taken, they should be recorded, preferably with action lines in the minutes, for example:

Extract from the minutes of practice meeting 3.7.89, Doddery Health Centre.

Item 4. The double yellow lines outside the surgery are being constantly abused; access is getting very difficult.

Action. Dr Crepit will write to the Traffic Superintendent to ask for increased vigilance and report back to the meeting in two months.

The practice manager may choose to keep her own record of the proceedings, but she is not the automatic choice for minute taker. She will be closely involved in the discussions. In any case, most practices have perfectly good shorthand secretaries. The minutes should be circulated immediately after the meeting so that those with action lines have a chance to act and so that errors can be notified.

Who is to be invited

We are not discussing here the sort of practice meeting where doctors discuss clinical cases in detail and make clinical decisions about individual patients, but about business meetings. A general rule might be to invite any one who might have a viewpoint.

The content of the meeting

The business meeting has two components. The first is concerned with delivery of care and the second with administration. Thus an agenda might look like this:

Doddery Health Centre Practice Meeting 4.7.89

Agenda
1 Minutes of the last meeting.
2 Matters arising from the last meeting.
3 The new diabetic clinic (Dr Old).
4 On call rota for bank holidays (Mrs Frail).
5 Parking outside surgery (Dr Crepit).
6 Any other business.

Delivery of care

In considering new ventures in the delivery of care and reviewing the way in which old patterns of care work, it is useful to place them into a pattern. Structure, process and outcome is a useful and convenient classification. The following example illustrates this.

Antenatal care at Doddery Health Centre

Structure	*Process*	*Outcome*
Antenatal clinic every Monday, 2.30 pm. Doctor and midwife present.	Urine, BP and weight taken by midwife, then see doctor. Object is to detect early problems.	75% of expectant mothers attend. Lowest infant death rate in region.

In this way the practice can look at what they are doing together in any field of care and see if the results (outcome) make it worthwhile. In this example it clearly is but if only half of the women had turned up the practice could ask why? Is the clinic at the wrong time? Are expectant mothers with children meeting other children from school at that time? (Structure) Do patients have to wait too long at the clinic? Do we need more staff available then to ease the flow through the clinic? Should the midwife see half or more of them completely? (Process)

Deconstructing a problem in the delivery of care like this simplifies it. It often produces a breakthrough in the muddled consideration of a problem that results from having been lost in it for a long time.

Administrative matters

These may appear straightforward, but are not always so. Within whose remit does an issue fall? Who will be delegated to handle it? Will the delegate be given authroity to see it through, and have his or her decision respected at the end? These are the issues that corrupt management, and the risks are high. If a proper mandate to deal with a problem is not transferred the delegate feels lessened and is less able to deal with it. If there is a risk of a decision being changed by one who sees him or herself as senior then the delegate risks fudging the issue and reaching a poorer solution in an attempt to satisfy too many people. Issues like these should be clarified at the meeting. 'If I make out a rota for the bank holidays for this year, do I have your guarantee that you will abide by it . . . ? Thank you, that has been minuted.'

Rotas

Rotas are a fair way of sharing work. Rotas can be useful in all sorts of situations apart from obvious ones like on-call duty and afternoons off. Here are some examples.

- Chairman of the practice meetings.
- Clinic duties (e.g. antenatal clinics).
- Afternoons off.
- On-call evenings.
- On-call for 'late calls'.
- Management liaison.
- Holiday cover.

Rotas do two things. They say 'today it is your turn to do the clinic, I'm busy upstairs with some writing.' and, just as importantly, 'Now it is my turn to get familiar with the way the practice is managed; you did it all last year.' Disputes are minimized and no one person hogs the job he or she likes at the expense of others. As stated, doctors benefit from discipline.

Other skills

The tools described will enable the practice manager to negotiate many of the difficulties she will experience in the interface between her and the doctor. She will be able to point to an established procedure for the resolution of difficulties and disputes. For some others, though, she will need more skills. Faced with personality conflicts, complaints against a doctor or a sick doctor, there are greater difficulties whose power to evoke emotion and prejudice will test the whole practice.

Personality conflicts

Doctors, being people, sometimes dislike each other. Social mores being what they are, it is difficult to express those feelings overtly, in a healthy way, but instead the opponents pursue a series of games, a guerrilla war, in which each vies with the other for the higher ground. This conflict, in which each suffers defeats and wins spurious victories, is distressing to watch for the outsider. Worse, though, it impinges on the whole practice and on the staff of the practice. Low morale follows quickly. Where is the role for the practice manager here? When the ongoing conflict threatens the clinical care of patients, directly through arguments over rotas and responsibility, or indirectly because progress cannot be made in the practice because of the blocking manoeuvres each employs, then the practice manager has a right to intervene. But each of the opponents has allies or sympathizers, and it may be that the practice manager herself is sympathetic to one point of view. How then can a solution be arrived at?

Covert tactics which do not state the real case are unhealthy. The current dispute, one of many, may have nothing to do with the original one; it is actually unlikely to do so. The dispute may be, indeed, not based on any clear ground, but on prejudice, e.g. one opponent may want to say, 'I hate the way he dresses; he never wears a tie in the surgery!', while his enemy states, 'he's the very antithesis of modern practice; look at his clothes.'

When games are being played, in the place of honesty, one solution is to expose the game for what it is. The whole practice has an interest in this, since their livelihoods are threatened by it. The place for the exposure has to be the practice meeting, or a specially called practice meeting, where the difficulties caused by the conflict can be aired. Those involved in the game are sometimes unaware of the disorder they cause. Putting it on the line, showing how it is damaging, is the first step to making it better. Showing it up for what it is, a squabble, allows the opponents to rethink, to try a better way. This is dangerous ground, risky to contemplate, yet the risk of allowing it to continue is worse. Like the abscess that festers away beneath the skin, it will eventually burst, probably incompletely and inconveniently. Better to lance it now, so it can heal cleanly and quickly.

The practice manager will not be alone in wanting the dispute over, for better or for worse. She will find allies, so that when the item appears on the special agenda, it will have the backing of many, not just one. Actions like this do not always win friends. The practice manager will need to learn that it is not always possible to be friendly with all or even any of the doctors. Friendships can be manipulative and, again, corrupt the good manager. Her interest is always for the well-being of the practice.

Complaints

Patients do complain about their treatemnt, or the doctor's manner, or the availability or otherwise of care. Because we all hate direct conflict, as we have seen, the complaint is not always addressed to the doctor. Commonly it is referred to the staff, the receptionists or the practice manager, with the anticipation that they will pass it on. Complaints can be frivolous, e.g. 'I've had to wait 20 minutes to see him; why is he always late?', in which case an explanation suffices; the patient has complained, heard the truth and, satisfied, departs. But what about more serious complaints? The following example illustrates this:

> I rang up three times last night to ask Dr Old to visit our lad. He's been ill with a pain in his tummy for a week; Dr Old said he'd see him in the morning surgery but he wouldn't come out when he'd had it for so long already. He said to give him Calpol and put him to bed. Well we did that but he was worse so we took him to the hospital and they kept him in. It's not right . . . '

You know that Dr Old is clearly in breach of his terms of service, yet what you don't know is Dr Old's version of the story. The course of action, then, is clear. You will pass on the patient's complaint to Dr Old. He will deal with it as he sees best, since clinical care is his responsibility. The outcome is only the concern of the practice manager insofar as she must not act to prejudice that outcome. She is not in a position to discuss the rights or wrongs with the patient and any attempt to do so would be prejudicial. But what about when the patient returns with the intention of making a formal complaint. Is it the duty of the practice manger to inform the patient about the procedure for complaints to the FHSA? To fail to do so looks defensive, and is, and runs the risk of the loss of all the remaining goodwill between the practice and the patient. To co-operate looks like collusion. To whom is your responsibility? The responsibility of the practice manager is to the doctors, the staff and the patients, to the whole practice. It is not to any one individual. The practice could have a complaints procedure which is laid out in the practice leaflet.

Sick doctors

Sometimes when patients complain, it is not directed at an aspect of clinical care, but about the way in which care was delivered. In this way many insights have come to light which have sometimes eluded staff with whom a doctor deals all day. Sadly, sometimes patients report that a doctor 'seemed drunk in the surgery today', and other matters come to light; 'he seems too irritable to be bothered most of the time now. He never used to be like that.' Patients often take staff into their confidence from knowing them over a long period when doctors have come and gone. Staff notice patterns of care too; a doctor starts losing his regulars to another partner. A doctor is persistently late. These, then, may be pointers to the biggest problem a practice can face, the alcoholic or drug abusing doctor. What is the role of the practice manger in this sad event? To restate the case for her role, she has a responsibility to the whole practice; its staff, its patients and its doctor. Indeed, the case for intervention is even clearer than in the case of patient complaints about clinical matters, because there the doctor can only lose by the exposure of the complaint, whereas here the doctor, now ill, stands a chance of gaining.

Once one statement is made about such a problem it is commonly found that many others have noticed a problem too. Again, human nature, fearing the consequences of exposure, conceals a problem, using that most potent of defences, denial. 'He can't be, he's always been wonderful with the patients.' Yet the truth is now evident. The practice manager, often the first to know, now has to decide on the best way to broach it. The options are: to talk to that doctor, talk to another doctor, or to talk to someone outside. Sadly, there are no absolutes, except that it has to be broached somewhere.

Talking to the doctor seems ideal, and honest, yet the practice manager needs to make her own judgment about her ability to do so, when she has weighed up her previous relationship with the doctor. Talking to another doctor seems disloyal, and may only foment gossip, if that doctor feels unable to deal with it. 'Someone outside' is the BMA contact telephone number for sick doctors, a confidential contact point for people in just this situation. The BMA simply contacts the sick doctor, via an intermediary, and offers help. There is no risk of referral to the GMC, this is purely a service offering help to sick doctors. It is wholly confidential and the sick doctor is under no obligation to take up the offer of help. No information is given to the doctor about whence the referral came.

Of course, not all sick doctors get better. It is also unusual for the issue not to come to a head if they do not. The practice manager has little control over what the outcome is, but does have a responsibility to initiate some action because her responsibility is to the whole practice.

Many of the scenarios above will be familiar to managers. Indeed many of the situations, e.g. disputes over who does what and how and when, illness and complaints are not unique to doctors. The tools for dealing with them in other groups are just the same. However, the other interfaces also have problems that are special.

The interface with office staff

The days have passed when staff members were all receptionists of one sort or another. Now a whole range of staff with different skills are employed by practices. A large practice might have records staff, computer staff, as well as receptionists. There may be a hierarchy of managers, at the top of which stands the practice manger, by virtue of her special skills. Indeed she may not share any of the skills of the office staff; her skill is in a different area which is to ensure the smooth running of the practice. Thus the twin problems of authority and seniority rear their heads. Many staff may have been longer in the practice than the manager. Some may have wanted her job! But the manager does not want to do other peoples' jobs. She has her own, and part of that job is to ensure that everyone is doing their job and only their job. She will use a tool for this part.

Job descriptions

The importance of a job description is described elsewhere in this book. Employees should be taken on on the basis of a job description set out earlier to fulfil a practice need. The FHSA will need this evidence in considering the question of reimbursement for the post, but much more importantly the employee must know what he or she is employed to do. In that way the employee knows when he or she is taking on extra work and the manager can decide if that is because someone else is not doing their job or because the job description was incomplete.

Staff meetings

The manager must have a forum for discussion with the office staff. Informal contacts will take place, as with the doctors, but the proper place for discussion about practice matters is a meeting which should, as with the doctors, have an agenda, be advertised and minuted. The meeting is an opportunity for communication in both directions, from manager to staff and vice versa. Further, this is an opportunity to plan, e.g. the institution of a new diabetic clinic, and discuss how this new work will be allocated. This may mean a change in a job description to be agreed and formalized.

Training and appraisal

The importance of training and appraisal is discussed in Chapter 3. Who will appraise the practice manager? There are options; the doctor, outsiders (other managers). It is up to the practice to decide who does it, but it must be done.

The interface with other members

Practice nurse

The practice will be running an appointments system for the nurse. Good liaison is essential to ensure that time is allocated appropriately for the different procedures. How will the nurse fit into the meetings going on in the practice? Should she be attending some, or all of them? The old guidelines apply; if the nurse can contribute or needs to learn from a meeting, then she should be there.

Others

Social workers, health visitors, district nurses, are in contact with the practice on a day-to-day basis. How does the manager ensure good communication in the practice? Are messages always delivered? If she is to keep the goodwill of all who come into contact with the practice, and ensure that the patients get the best deal, communication systems are essential. They are the responsibility of the practice manager, and are discussed fully in the previous chapter.

Conclusion

Much of the work of the practice manager involves entering others' territory to ensure the smooth running of the practice. The division of labour is her responsibility, and the negotiation that ensues is challenging. The use of the tools we have seen ensures that all parties are satisfied with the outcome.

6 Personnel Management of Practice Staff

The law and employment

THIS section is designed to help practice managers see the connections between employment law and their day-to-day practice in dealing with employees. It takes the reader through various stages in the employment relationship. It suggests the good practices that might be adopted and draws attention to the rights of individual employees. Hopefully, it enables practice managers to see the role of employment law in a constructive and practical way and *not* as a threat or a difficulty.

Some practice managers may feel that employment law has only slight relevance to their own situation. They may work in small medical practices. Nevertheless, they should read through this section in order to identify those key parts of legislation that may affect them.

Obviously, it has not been possible to cover in great detail all aspects of statutory employment rights. This section is very much an initial guide. If any practice manager needs more detailed information, the next recommended step is to obtain the free set of guides published by the Department of Employment. (These are generally available at Department of Employment offices, Job Centres, and Citizens Advice Bureaux.) The standard work in general practice is *Employing Staff* by Norman Ellis, published by the British Medical Journal. It will also be helpful to obtain the advisory handbook, *Discipline at Work*, published by the Advisory, Conciliation and Arbitration Service, and available free from ACAS, 27 Wilton Street, London SW1 7AZ.

Recruiting staff

Introduction

When staff are being recruited to any job, whether it is a full-time, part-time or temporary post, it is important to carry out the process properly. It creates a good impression of the organization if prospective staff are treated well. It can make a newly-recruited person feel well-motivated to their new job. Above all, it helps ensure that standards set in law are obeyed.

The law that relates to the recruitment and appointment of staff:

1 outlaws discrimination and aims to promote equal opportunity;
2 requires certain employers to recruit a percentage of disabled people;
3 protects young people;
4 outlines the contractual information that the employee must have.

This section will consider the various stages that are likely to be taken in recruiting a new employee. Practice managers will see how, at each stage, the law sets a standard of expected behaviour. The purpose of the law in this process is essentially derived from 'good employment practice'. The law should not be seen as an obstacle. If it is integrated into the way staff are recruited, it should help practice managers organize both themselves and the employment relationship much more satisfactorily.

The stages involved in recruiting staff are:

- producing a job description, title and requirements;
- producing a person specification;
- deciding on whether the job is full-time, part-time or temporary;
- advertising the post;
- providing an application form;
- holding selection interview(s);
- sending a letter of appointment;
- agreeing a contract of employment;
- providing written details of certain conditions of employment.

Job descriptions, titles and person specifications

A job description principally involves deciding the main purpose of the job; the tasks that an employer expects will be undertaken; the degree of responsibility an employee will have and the standards of performance to be reached by the employee. Linked with this, an employer will decide whether the job is full-time, part-time (and for how many hours per week) or temporary (and, if so, for how long).

A person specification principally involves deciding the attributes of the person who is to fill the job. These specifications can be very complex for some jobs. Broadly speaking, they may cover physique, gender, health, appearance, attainments, general intelligence and special aptitudes. In considering these aspects of recruitment, practice managers must take account of the provisions of the discrimination legislation and that relating to disability.

The three main sets of legislation in this area are:

1 the Disabled Persons (Employment) Acts of 1944 and 1958;
2 the Sex Discrimination Acts of 1975 and 1986;
3 the Race Relations Act of 1976.

The requirements on disability are unlikely to affect many medical practices *directly*. The law requires that employers with more than 20 employees recruit 3% of their workforce from the register of disabled persons maintained by the Department of Employment. Very few practices will have this number of employees. Nevertheless, practice managers ought to think positively. Whilst the law requires certain employers to meet standards of good practice, it does not prevent employers outside this category from approaching the recruitment of disabled people in a constructive and humane way.

A *Code of Good Practice on the Employment of Disabled People* (published originally in 1984, and available from the Department of Employment) proposes the following approach for employers.

Box 6.1: Good practice on employment of disabled people

- Have an open mind on jobs which disabled people can do, even with a quite severe handicap. Draw up and assess job requirements in as unrestrictive a way as possible when vacancies occur. Be prepared to make minor modifications.
- Look at what disabled people can do rather than at their disability when considering them for jobs. Avoid the assumption that disabled people are going to cause problems. Look realistically at any handicap that may arise in specific job situations.
- Assess job and career prospects flexibly. Bear in mind that disabled people may be able to do jobs differently from other workers without loss of effectiveness. Consider, for example, the use of special aids or the re-structuring of the job tasks.

The Sex Discrimination and Race Relations legislation have a much more wide-ranging effect on these early stages of defining job descriptions and person specifications. Both pieces of legislation have broadly similar provisions. They are applicable to all employers, irrespective of size, so even a small medical practice is covered by them.

Generally, these Acts outlaw those 'person specifications' which include requirements for a post-holder to be, for example male or female; single or married; black or white. This would clearly be contrary to the '*direct discrimination*' provisions. However, there are certain limited circumstances in which it is permissible to specify an employee's gender or ethnic origin or marital status. Two exempted categories, for example, are those covering 'decency or privacy' (e.g. lavatory cleaners); and those where 'personal services' promoting welfare can 'most effectively' be provided by a person of a particular gender or ethnic origin (*see* Fig. 6.1). (In these circumstances, then, the law allows an employer to designate a person's gender or ethnic origin as an 'occupational qualification', provided it is a '*genuine* occupational qualification'.)

```
┌─────────────────────────────────────────────┐
│         SHORT STAY YOUNG HOMELESS            │
│              PROJECT LTD                      │
│              wish to appoint                  │
│                                               │
│          A BLACK MALE                        │
│          HOSTEL WORKER                       │
│                                               │
│  for our multi-racial short-stay hostel for  │
│  young men and women in Bina Gardens,         │
│  South Kensington.                            │
│                                               │
│  The hostel provides accommodation for 27    │
│  residents and attempts to help them find     │
│  suitable long-term places. The job can be    │
│  both frustrating and stimulating and         │
│  requires sensitivity, flexibility, a sense   │
│  of humour and a strong commitment to equal   │
│  opportunities.                               │
│                                               │
│  Salary £10,956 pa (inc. LW) plus sleep-in    │
│  payments.                                    │
│                                               │
│  For further details and application form     │
│  telephone Maria Duda on 01-272 8089.         │
│  Closing date: January 30, 1988.              │
│                                               │
│  Section 7 (2) (e) Sex Discrimination Act     │
│  applies.                                     │
│  Section 5 (2) (e) Race Relations Act         │
│  applies.                                     │
└─────────────────────────────────────────────┘
```

Figure 6.1

In addition to direct discrimination, the law also identifies '*indirect discrimination*'. It is a more subtle form of bias and occurs effectively where a condition or requirement is applied to a job which is not directly relevant to the job and, therefore, has an adverse effect on the numbers of, for example, men or women, or black or white people who are able to meet the requirement. The bias may be unintended. The practices may appear fair, as between men and women, but the employment practice may be discriminatory in operation and in effect (*see* Box 6.2).

Box 6.2: Age discrimination and women

In 1977, the Civil Service age rule was successfully complained against. The Civil Service had stated that candidates for the post of executive officer should be aged between 17½ and 28 years. The Employment Appeals Tribunal held that fewer women aged 25 to 35 years could comply *in practice* with an age limit of 28 than could men. This was because a large proportion of women at this age were preoccupied with child-bearing and child-rearing at this time. Mrs Price, the complainant, was 36 years and married with children.

Another form of indirect discrimination that practice managers should be aware of relates to qualifications for a job and also the issue of language proficiency. It is possible, for example, to overstate the standards required. A lowering of standards is not advocated, but, practice managers should ask themselves 'What qualifications and language skills do I *realistically* want from a person undertaking a particular job?' In this way, people from different ethnic backgrounds are then less likely to be discriminated against.

It is essential to remember, insofar as indirect discrimination is concerned, that an employer has to *justify* the employment practice. There is no clear legal definition of justifiability. An employer must be able to show that an employment practice is *necessary in a reasonable and commonsense way*. It would be a good idea for a practice manager to ask herself, for example: 'What is the *effect* of our recruitment practices? Do they, in the way they operate, discriminate against particular groups? What might we do to change them?'

Employment status

Jobs may be organized in terms of length of working time to meet the operational needs of an employer. They may be full-time, part-time, or temporary. Also, a useful and growing type of employment relationship is job share—where two individuals share a full-time job on two part-time contracts.

The principal way in which the law relates to employment status is through the right of a person to complain about an infringement of their employment rights. As far as gender and race discrimination issues are concerned, any employee, irrespective of employment status or length of service has an immediate right of complaint to an Industrial Tribunal. In relation to other aspects of employment law (e.g. dismissal, and information about the contract of employment) there are variations to these rights. (These are outlined in the section 'How employees enforce their rights'.)

Advertising a job

There are two aspects to this part of the recruitment process that practice managers need to be aware of in terms of the law: the advertisement itself; and where it is placed. The advertisement should generally be encouraging to a wide range of potential applicants and therefore might include not only a statement that the organization is an equal opportunities employer but also a more specific statement (*see* Box 6.3). This is a reflection of 'positive action' (which, unlike positive discrimination, is lawful). Through this an employer makes positive steps to encourage under-represented groups to apply for particular jobs.

Box 6.3: Positive action

As part of the Council's equal opportunity employment policy applications are invited from people regardless of race, creed, nationality, disability, age, sex or responsibility for children or dependants and from lesbians and gay men.

* * * * * *

This authority positively welcomes applicants from all sections of the community, and particularly those presently under-represented, people from ethnic minority groups, people with disabilities, and for post graded Scale 5 and above—women.

As indicated earlier, job titles must be non-sexist. The way advertisements are worded must not imply that people of a particular gender or ethnic group are required (unless, as mentioned above, the 'genuine occupational qualification' provision is appropriate).

The location of advertisements is particularly important—not just in terms of equal opportunities policies but also to enable employers to obtain the best response. To meet both these objectives, then, it is advisable to choose a widely-read newspaper. Practice managers might probably consider local free newspapers for many of the jobs they recruit for. If there are local ethnic or women's periodicals, consider these also. Apart from the equal opportunities implications, it is sensible if a medical practice is in an area where there are shortages of potential recruits, to extend advertising in this way.

One type of 'advertising' that some employers use—often because it is seen as cost-effective—is *'word of mouth' recruitment*. The main drawback to this type of recruitment is that it may indirectly discriminate against groups not currently represented in the workforce. If a practice manager does use this method, then she should ask herself two questions.

- Is it discriminatory in effect in our practice? (i.e. are we failing to attract under-represented groups like black women, for example, from the local labour market?)

- Does it provide a wide enough range of suitable applicants for a proper selection to be made? (i.e. are we 'missing out' on potentially good applicants?)

There is then, clearly, both a legal and a practical aspect to this recruitment method.

Application form

Practice managers may not use application forms. If you do (and it is perhaps good practice to have a simple one) then think carefully about the information needed. Often employers ask for information on age, marital status, and number of children, for example, which can be merely intrusive and of no importance when considering a person's suitability for a job. Such questions contravene the spirit of discrimination legislation. The information an employer *needs to know* relates to a person's qualifications, experience and ability to meet the specified tasks of the job.

Interviewing applicants

Although personnel management experts, rightly, have reservations about the value of the interview, it is still the most commonly used selection tool. It serves two purposes.

1   It can help make some assessment of an applicant's capacity and motivation to do a particular job. It is especially useful when trying to assess a person's impact on others and their general disposition. (It is less useful in assessing intelligence and special aptitudes.)
2   It can help the applicant form his/her own assessment of the job and the organization.

The outcome of the selection process will only be satisfactory if both the applicant and the practice manager have felt that the process was handled fairly. Consequently, considerable importance must be attached to the questions asked in the interview. These should relate primarily to the person's ability to do the job, to their experience, to the skills they have developed, and (possibly) to their preparedness to train and develop new skills. It can again be intrusive and possibly evidence of indirect discrimination to question, for example, a woman about her domestic arrangements and circumstances.

It would be fair for a practice manager, therefore, to ask applicants if they could meet all the conditions required to do the job (including attendance at particular designated times). But, generally, it is against the spirit and intention of the law to say: 'How many children do you have? What do you do about them if they are sick?' The Equal Opportunities Commission, in a model equal opportunities policy, says: 'It is not discriminatory to ask questions about such matters as applicants' home commitments, *but* where such questions are asked it is important to explain the reasons for asking them, to ask them in a way in which they can reasonably be answered, to ask similar questions of *all* candidates, and to relate the answer *purely to the job requirements*'.

An offer of appointment

Once the selection process is finished, an offer of appointment is normally then made to one of the applicants. This can be done either verbally (often at the end of the interviews) or in a letter.

If a verbal offer is made, then make note of what is said at the time and make sure that all details are quickly confirmed in a letter. It is normal, when offering a job, to tell the person the starting date, the hours of work, the place of work, their rate of pay, and perhaps, the employer's agreement to any special arrangements (e.g. that the new employee can take a pre-booked holiday and that this might be without pay). An employer may also have indicated the existence of a sick pay scheme and a pension scheme (and any special aspects relating to that individual). All this information is particularly important because it clearly relates to the new employee's contract of employment.

The contract of employment

In law, the whole issue of the contract of employment is very complex. But, there are certain practical steps that can be taken by practice managers. These should help minimize any likely difficulties.

A contract of employment is a promise, freely arrived at, that can be enforced in the courts. It is agreed between the individual employee and the employer. It is usually of indefinite duration (although, obviously, it can be for any fixed period, e.g. a month, three months, a year). It may be in writing, it may be agreed verbally, or (and most often) it may be part verbal and part in writing.

The main sources of an employee's contract of employment are usually:

- conditions of employment indicated by the employer verbally or in the letter of appointment or staff handbook;
- agreements about pay and conditions between trade unions and employers;
- custom and practice;
- various implied terms.

Information about what is contained in the contract of employment of certain employees must be given to them within 13 weeks of their starting employment (*see* next section on 'Written statements'). To find the contract of employment of any individual employee, then, it will be necessary to explore these four areas.

Employer-determined conditions may cover hours worked, overtime and shift arrangements, holidays, sick pay scheme, notice, pensions, pay scales, and arrangements for payments to be made. It may cover many aspects of the job, particular to a specific job or organization (e.g. confidentiality).

Negotiated agreements in unionized organizations often cover many of the issues just mentioned. The provisions of these agreements relevant to each individual is 'incorporated' (i.e. included) in each individual's contract of employment.

Although collective agreements in themselves are usually voluntary agreements, i.e. not legally enforceable, the provisions relating to each individual become legally enforceable (in respect of that individual) because of the process of 'incorporation'. It is important to remember that even where there is a negotiated agreement in an organization, it is also likely to be supplemented by some employer-determined conditions in areas not covered by the agreement.

Custom and practice usually refers to long-standing working practices. They can be contractually binding if they are widely known about, reasonable, and the individual employee knows for certain the effect of the custom on them as an individual.

Implied terms are part of an individual's contract of employment that derives from law. An employer has to meet certain obligations, for example:

- he must pay an employee's wages or salary;
- he must not make unauthorized deductions from an employee's pay packet. There is a statutory requirement to deduct income tax and national insurance contributions. Apart from these, an employer must obtain the employee's consent for deductions, e.g. pension contributions, union subs, attachment of earnings orders made by courts for the payment of fines and maintenance. If an employer proposes, for example, to deduct money for some loss (breakage or shortage from a till) then, it must be clear in the initial contract of employment that this deduction is liable to be made. (The Wages Act 1986 sets a limit to the proportion of such deductions that can be made in the retail trade);
- he must provide safe systems of work. This obligation is elaborated by the Health and Safety at Work Act 1974 and supplementary regulations and legislation;
- he must obey the law.

Likewise, an employee has to meet certain general obligations for example:

- he/she must obey all lawful and reasonable instructions;
- he/she must co-operate with the employer in fulfilling a legal duty;
- he/she must take reasonable care (it is possible for the employer to claim compensation if he sustains loss because of the employee's negligence);
- he/she must be trustworthy.

Employees are rarely, if ever, told about implied terms. But, nevertheless, they exist and can be invoked. They cover, as it can be seen, some very important obligations on both parties.

The information given to employees about the contract of employment varies very widely. Some (primarily full-time permanent employees) may receive highly detailed written documentation and/or a staff handbook. Some other employees (particularly temporary and many part-time workers) may receive little or nothing in writing.

The law says that certain categories of employee *must* receive, as a minimum, a written statement of particular main terms and conditions in the contract of employment.

The written statement of terms and conditions

This must be provided within 13 weeks of an employee starting employment to the following employees: (i) those employees who normally work 16 hours or more per week; and (ii) those who work between 8 and 16 hours and have 5 years service. If an employee does not receive this information then he/she may complain to an Industrial Tribunal. Obviously, any employer adopting 'good employment practice' will provide such information to *all* employees irrespective of employment status or length of service.

Under the Employment Protection (Consolidation) Act 1978, the following information should be given.

1 The *names* of the employer and the employee.
2 The *date employment began* and an indication of whether any employment with a previous employer counts as part of the employee's continuous employment. (Length of service is particularly important in relation to, for example, notice entitlement and the provisions of sick pay schemes and pension arrangements.)
3 The *job title* (but a job description is not required).
4 The scale or rate of *remuneration*; or the method of calculating remuneration (including any commission, bonus, overtime). Remuneration covers *all* forms of pay.
5 *How often a person is paid*—whether it is weekly, monthly or at some other interval.

6   *Hours* of work (e.g. 35 hours per week) and normal working hours each day.

7   Entitlement of annual *holidays*, holiday pay and public holidays.

8   Conditions relating to *sickness* or injury, including provisions for sick pay.

9   Conditions relating to *pensions* and pension schemes.

10 The length of *notice* to terminate the contract that the employee is obliged to give and is entitled to receive. If the contract is for a fixed term (e.g. for a temporary worker on a three-month contract), indicate the date the contract expires. (Notice entitlement is covered in more detail in the section 'Ending the contract'.)

11 Specify any *disciplinary rules* which apply to the employee, and the person to whom the employee can appeal against any disciplinary decision (*see* section on 'Handling staff'). This requirement does *not* now apply to those employers who have less than 20 employees. However, practice managers may feel that it would be good practice to inform employees of these disciplinary arrangements.

12 Indicate the name of a person who will deal with *grievances* and the procedure to be followed.

Sometimes, there are *no* agreed terms under some of these headings (e.g. sick pay, or pensions). If this is the case, the written statement should say so.

Under some of the headings (e.g. discipline, grievances, pensions) a long and detailed procedure may exist. It is not necessary to provide a copy for each employee, provided they are told where they may have reasonable access to see the documents.

Practice managers might like to have a standard form produced along the following lines (*see* Box 6.4). This could then be easily completed for every new employee. If existing employees do not have this information, then they should be given it.

One final set of information that employees should receive regularly is an *itemized pay statement*. Every pay statement must give the following particulars:

- the gross amount of wages or salary;
- the amounts of any fixed deductions and the purposes for which they are made;
- the amounts of any variable deductions and the purposes for which they are made;
- the net amount of wages or salary payable;
- the amount and method of each part-payment when different parts of the net amount are paid in different ways.

Complaints about the non-provision of an itemized pay statement can be made to an Industrial Tribunal.

Box 6.4: Statement of main terms and conditions of employment

This statement is provided under the provisions of the Employment Protection (Consolidation) Act 1978.

NAME OF EMPLOYER
NAME OF EMPLOYEE
DATE EMPLOYMENT BEGAN

1   You are employed as a (insert job title).
2   You will work . . . . hours per week; your hours of work will be . . . . . .
3   You will be paid £ . . . . . per week/or £ . . . . . per hour.
4   You are entitled to . . . . days holiday per year. This will be paid at your normal earnings rate. (If employees are entitled to more holidays according to length of service this can also be stated.)
5   If you are unable to work because of sickness, the following arrangements apply: . . . . (If it is a very detailed scheme, then the employee could be referred to a document held by the practice manager or on display in the practice on a staff noticeboard.)   (If there is no scheme, say there is none.)
6   Your pension arrangements are set out in . . . . (mention a handbook or some other document which is available from the practice manager).
    (If there is no appropriate pension scheme, say there is none.)
7   *Either*
    If you wish to terminate your employment, you must give. . . . . weeks notice.
    You are entitled to receive the following notice from your employer . . . . . . (see the statutory minimum rights in section 'Ending the contract').

    Or

    Your contract is for a fixed term and will end on . . . .
8   Disciplinary rules and procedures are available from the practice manager or on display in the practice.
9   If you have a grievance about any employment issue, raise it with . . . . (name).   If you are not satisfied with their answer then you can appeal to . . . . (name).

Handling staff

Introduction

There are a number of important aspects of the day-to-day employment relationship that are influenced by the law. This section will therefore, comment on the following:

- appraising employees;
- the development, training and promotion of employees;
- the provision of rewards and benefits;
- rights to time off;
- discipline and dismissal;
- sick absence and ill health;
- varying the contract of employment.

In considering these issues, it is important to remember that the law on discrimination in employment runs as a thread through these aspects of the employment relationship. The issues of direct and indirect discrimination, mentioned in the section 'Recruiting staff', are as relevant here. In addition, there is a growing body of law affecting the question of equal pay. Also, there are extensive legal considerations relating to discipline and dismissal.

Appraising employees

Performance appraisal can be a very useful management tool. It need not be limited to large organizations. It can be beneficial also for small organizations to review the performance of individual employees. This could be undertaken on a regular (six-monthly or annual) basis, through a formal, recorded interview.

The aspects of performance appraisal that a practice manager might like to consider as helpful are:

- a review of an individual's performance set against the employee's job description and the expectations of the standards of performance indicated by management;
- a review of the employee's skills and the extent to which they might be developed or are under-utilized;
- an identification of a person's training needs, of (further) counselling needed, and of the quality of supervision they receive;
- a consideration of the employee's own expectations about their job, their role in the organization, and the effect of other staff on the way they work.

It is important to remember two aspects of the law when considering the way in which appraisal might be operated. First of all, do not see appraisal as a part of the disciplinary process. The purpose is not to punish. It is to review performance honestly and to promote any required improvement. Practice managers, therefore, need to make the purpose of these interviews clear at the start.

Secondly, performance appraisal needs to be seen in the context of fair treatment. It should be seen as a way of developing employees and, wherever possible, as a means to promotion and further development. This should be clearly set within an equal opportunities context.

The development, training and promotion of employees

Large organizations often develop sophisticated schemes for employee development. Even in a small organization, like a medical practice, development and training should be an important consideration.

Practice managers might usefully identify three aspects:

- the training needs of existing staff in terms of skill development;
- the training and development opportunities that might be provided to enable certain staff to apply for promotions;
- the training needs of the practice manager herself.

Depending on the type of training needs identified, various courses can be provided or are already available. The Practice Manager Development Programme and the Practice Receptionist Programme are contributors to this provision. Organizations like the Industrial Society run other short courses and workshops; and the Institute of Personnel Management might also advise as can AMSPAR, AHCPA and the RCGP.

Employment law affects training in one particular way—under equal opportunities legislation. Under 'positive action', an employer is encouraged to ensure that under-represented groups are given specific access to training in order to assist in their development and promotion within an organization.

Rewards and benefits

The issue of discrimination in relation to the rewards and benefits for employees can be very complex. In this section a brief outline of the statutory provisions is set out. If a practice manager becomes involved in an Industrial Tribunal complaint, it is advisable to obtain specific professional advice.

The Equal Pay Act 1970 allows a woman to claim equal pay with men who are employed on 'like work' or 'work rated as equivalent' under a job evaluation scheme. So, if men collectively are paid more than the complainant for doing the same work, that is unlawful discrimination.

'Like work' is defined as being 'of the same or a broadly similar nature' providing that 'the differences (if any) between the things she (the complainant) does and the things they (the comparators) do are not of practical importance in relation to terms and conditions of employment' (e.g. in comparing clerks with clerks).

'Work rated as equivalent' is where 'her job and their job have been given an equal value, in terms of the demands made on the worker under various headings (for example, effort, skill, decision) on a study undertaken with a view to evaluating in those terms the jobs to be done by all or any of the employees in an undertaking' (i.e. jobs graded equally in a job evaluation system).

In 1982, it was determined by the European Court of Justice that Britain was 'in breach of the (European Communities 1975) directive in that women were not entitled to equal pay for work of equal value *unless* their employer had chosen to undertake a job evaluation study'. In fact, the original 1970 Act had actively *discouraged* companies from installing payment systems based on a job-evaluated grade structure so that they could remain immune from claims for equality under the 'work rated as equivalent' provision. So, from 1984, the Equal Pay (Amendment) Regulations (or 'Equal Value Regulations') came into force in Britain. These added a third condition under which a woman could claim equal pay with a man for 'work of equal value'. 'Work of equal value' is defined as being 'where a woman is employed on work which is, in terms of the demands made on her (for instance, under such headings as effort, skill and decision) of equal value to that of a man in the same employment'.

If a woman now complains to an Industrial Tribunal that her work is of equal value to that of a man (any one man) in the same organization, then, in the absence of a job evaluation system covering both jobs, 'equal value' is assessed by an *independent expert* appointed by the Tribunal. The expert examines and compares the two jobs in isolation using whatever factors are considered to be most relevant to these jobs. If the independent expert assesses the two jobs to be of equal value in this abstract context, then, assuming the man is paid more than the woman, discrimination on the grounds of sex is assumed to be occurring (or to have occurred) unless there is a valid reason (i.e. 'genuine material factor') involved.

The law covers rewards or benefits in other respects:

- time off for antenatal care;
- the right not to be dismissed for pregnancy;
- maternity leave and the right to return to work;
- maternity pay;
- the right to equal retirement ages.

Any pregnant woman, irrespective of length of service or employment status (e.g. full-time or part-time) is entitled to reasonable *time off work* with pay for antenatal care visits. A pregnant woman may also have a *right not to be dismissed* because of her pregnancy. The exceptions to this are:

- where her condition makes it impossible for her to do her job adequately;
- if it would be against the law for her to do her particular job whilst pregnant.

In such cases, the employer must, however, offer the employee a suitable alternative vacancy, if one is available (before or on the date when her employment is due to be terminated). If there is such a vacancy, but the employer fails to offer it to her, then her dismissal will be unfair.

The Employment Protection (Consolidation) Act 1978 does *not* give a right to maternity leave but rather a *right to return to work*. This latter right is subject to certain conditions. The key ones are:

- if the employee works for 16 hours per week or more, she must have at least two years service with the same employer immediately before the beginning of the 11th week before the expected week of confinement;
- if the employee works for eight to 16 hours per week, she must have five years service;
- the employee must notify her employer in writing, at least 21 days before her maternity absence begins, that she is having a baby, when it is expected and that she intends to return to work for her employer. (This must be done as early as reasonably possible if it is not done within the 21 days.);
- The employer has the right to send a written request to the employee, not earlier than 49 days from the date of confinement, asking her to confirm in writing that she intends to return. (The employee must reply in writing within 14 days of receiving the request, otherwise she may lose the right to return.);
- the employee must inform her employer of the date she proposes to return to work, in writing, at least 21 days before that date. (The date on which an employee returns to work is for her to decide, provided it is before the end of the period of 29 weeks beginning with the week in which her child is born subject of course to any considerations relating to illness.)

An employee's right to return to work may be restricted if the former job is no longer available because of redundancy, if the employee unreasonably refuses an offer of suitable alternative employment, or if the organization has five or less employees and it is not reasonably practicable for the employer to hold open the old job or offer suitable alternative employment.

An employee who satisfies certain conditions is entitled to receive *maternity pay* from her employer for the first six weeks of absence because of pregnancy. (The six weeks do not have to be taken in one unbroken period.) The key conditions are:

- if the employee works for 16 hours per week or more, she must have at least two years service with the same employer immediately before the beginning of the 11th week before the expected week of confinement;
- if the employee works for eight to 16 hours per week, she must have five years service;
- as far as is reasonably practicable, the employee should tell the employer at least 21 days before she stops work that she intends to do so because of her condition.

Broadly speaking, the amount of maternity pay due for each week is nine-tenths of a week's pay (as defined in the Act) less the amount of the flat-rate National Insurance maternity allowance (whether or not this is due in part or in full to the employee).

A new employment right for women was introduced in the Sex Discrimination Act of 1986. It is now unlawful for an employer to dismiss a woman who has reached the retiring age of 60 if men in that employment do not have to retire until 65 years. (This change in legislation arose from a successful appeal to the European Court of Justice by Miss Helen Marshall, a former senior dietitian employed by a health authority.)

Rights to time off

In the preceding section, the issue of time off work for antenatal care was considered. The law provides several other rights to time off, with or without pay, depending on the circumstances. In fact, the Employment Protection (Consolidation) Act 1978 talks of 'reasonable' time off. This means that the employer has to make a judgement about what is reasonable in the circumstances of each individual case. In making this decision, the employer can take account of the following:

- how much time off is required in general by the employee;
- how much time off is required on this particular occasion;
- how much time off the employee has already been permitted for this purpose and for other purposes;
- the circumstances of the employer's business (including its size) and the effect of the employee's absence upon it.

A statutory *right to time off with pay* exists for trade union representatives participating in industrial relations activities between their employer and their union; for union representatives undergoing union training courses; for employees who are being made redundant to enable them to look for alternative work. Pay can be defined as either average earnings or the normal earnings that employee would have received had they been working at that particular time. (The amount of money to be received is more predictable and easier to calculate where the employee is on a straight salary.)

A statutory *right to time off* exists for employees who are local magistrates, local authority councillors or members of a tribunal for example. While there is nothing to prevent an employer from making payment to an employee for time off for these public duties, there is no obligation to do so unless there is an agreement with an individual or their trade union.

Discipline and dismissal

The law provides two things to assist employers in this area:

1 a framework of law relating to 'fair dismissal'; and
2 a Code of Practice which provides guidance on the way in which disciplinary hearings should be handled.

Practice managers may feel that disciplinary issues may not involve them to the same extent as say a hospital or a local authority. To some degree, this is true. ACAS, in its advice on discipline, does recognize that small organizations have particular considerations. However, there are certain principles and practices that should be accepted by all organizations in their dealings with their staff.

The first point to consider is *the purpose of discipline*, as such. The word implies 'punishment'. Yet ACAS, in its Code of Practice (which has been approved by Parliament) says: 'Disciplinary procedures should not be viewed primarily as a means of imposing sanctions. They should also be designed to emphasize and encourage improvements in individual conduct'—and one might add, in standards of performance.

A good manager, then, wherever possible will aim to encourage improvements as a first step. This may involve counselling or advising the employee on what needs to be done; telling them how you, as a practice manager, expect them to behave or perform; and asking about any difficulties they may have in meeting these expectations.

To handle discipline, an employer needs two things: disciplinary rules and a disciplinary procedure. ACAS says that both are necessary for 'promoting fairness and order in the treatment of individuals and in the conduct of industrial relations. They also assist an organization to operate effectively'.

Disciplinary rules set a framework for employees' behaviour. They indicate, in large part, the employer's expectations. ACAS makes the point that 'the rules required will vary according to the particular circumstances such as the type of work, working conditions and the size of the establishment'.

Practice managers should review their existing rules: Are there any currently in operation whether in writing or not'? Would it be helpful to adopt some additional rules? The Code says: 'When drawing up rules the aim should be to specify clearly and concisely those necessary for efficient and safe performance of work and for the maintenance of satisfactory relations within the workforce and between employees and management. Rules should not be so general as to be meaningless'.

It was mentioned earlier in this textbook, when the contract of employment was being discussed, that employers should notify employees of the disciplinary rules. This is a right relating to the statement of written terms of employment. Obviously, if employees clearly know the rules in the workplace, then employers can fairly take action for breach of these rules (*see* Box 6.5).

Box 6.5: Disciplinary rules for small companies

As a minimum rules should:
- be simple, clear and in writing;
- be displayed prominently in the workplace;
- be known and fully understood by all employees;
- cover issues such as absence, timekeeping, health and safety and use of company facilities (add others relevant to your organization);
- indicate the type of conduct which will normally lead to disciplinary action other than dismissal examples may include persistent lateness or unauthorized absence;
- indicate the type of conduct which will normally lead to dismissal without notice—examples may include working dangerously, stealing or fighting, although much will depend on the circumstances of each offence.

A *disciplinary procedure* concerns the way in which an employer deals with disciplinary issues. It 'helps to ensure that the standards are adhered to and also provides a fair method of dealing with alleged failures to observe them'. At the end of the procedure a penalty may be given to the employee. The ACAS Code indicates various features of procedures, It is useful to consider these, particularly in relation to medical practices as small organizations. Procedures should:

1 be in writing;
2 specify which employees they apply to;
3 provide for matters to be dealt with quickly (this involves holding an *initial* hearing preferably within a working day of the alleged offence having been committed);

4   indicate the disciplinary actions which might be taken (these are discussed later);

5   specify the levels of management which have the authority to take the various forms of disciplinary action (obviously, in small organizations there are few levels in the managerial hierarchy, so, a practice manager will need to consider carefully those people, including herself, who can be responsible for particular disciplinary decisions—this is also discussed later);

6   provide for individual employees to be informed of the complaints against them and to be given an opportunity to state their case before any decisions are reached;

7   give the individual employee the right to be accompanied by a trade union representative or by a fellow worker of his/her choice (the practice manager should ensure that the employee is told of this right—even if the employee does not wish to exercise it);

8   ensure that disciplinary action is not taken until the case has been carefully investigated (normally by the practice manager);

9   ensure that individuals are given an explanation for any penalty imposed (this should normally be done by the practice manager)

10   provide a right of appeal and specify the procedure to be followed. (In medical practices, there may be few appeal levels. These normally relate to the levels of disciplinary authority mentioned in (5) above. This issue is discussed later. Practice managers should tell an employee of his/her right of appeal.)

None of these requirements impose any special difficulty for practice managers. They are requirements which, essentially, embody the principle of 'fair treatment'. The only requirement that may be significantly modified by workplace organization is (5)—i.e. that relating to the number of managerial levels.

Penalties against individual employees are considered in the Code of Practice. The range of penalties normally available to an employer are:

- an informal verbal warning;
- formal verbal warning;
- a written warning;
- a final written warning;
- dismissal with notice;
- dismissal without notice.

(An employer may, as a punishment, suspend an employee without pay or demote him/her. These are only lawful if they are provided for in that individual's contract of employment.)

Bearing in mind that a key purpose of disciplinary procedures is to encourage improvement, then an *informal verbal warning* from a supervisor may be sufficient. Basically, the supervisor is telling the individual to 'take more care' or 'don't do that again'. It is used for 'minor infringements' in terms of conduct or minor defects in standards of work.

Alternatively, a supervisor may feel that a *formal verbal warning* is more appropriate. This should be recorded (and retained for, perhaps, six months). If the issue is more serious, or there is persistent minor misconduct or poor performance, a *written warning* may be used. (This likewise may be retained on an employee's record for six to 12 months.)

A *final written warning* can be used where there is persistent misconduct or poor performance or, alternatively, where a disciplinary offence has been committed that is so serious that a person is close to being dismissed. This written warning 'should contain a statement that any recurrence would lead to suspension or dismissal or some other penalty, as the case may be'.

The final penalty available to an employer is dismissal. The ACAS Code says: 'ensure that, except for gross misconduct, no employees are dismissed for a first breach of discipline'.

If an employee is dismissed for serious, or gross, misconduct (such as theft, assault, harassment) then it can be—and may well be—*without notice*. This is sometimes referred to as 'summary dismissal'. It means that an employer can sack a person straight away (but, obviously, after a disciplinary investigation and hearing) without any regard to their length of service or their entitlement to notice (*see* later section on 'Ending the contract').

Usually, if an employee is dismissed it is a result of persistent misconduct (e.g. lateness) or persistent poor performance. Such an employee may have had a series of verbal and written warnings. The dismissal then may be *with notice* (i.e. the amount of notice that the individual employee is entitled to receive in view of their length of service). However, if the employer wishes the employee to go immediately after the disciplinary hearing, then it is lawful to give the employee his/her appropriate pay instead of notice (e.g. one month's pay in lieu of one month's notice).

A question that inevitably concerns managers is: *which managers are entitled to impose these disciplinary penalties?* This, inevitably, relates to the issue of the managerial structure mentioned earlier. Assuming a large medical practice, then the disciplinary responsibilities might be allocated as follows.

Senior partner (GP)

- Dismissal (instant or with notice).
- Hearing appeal on disciplinary warnings.

Practice manager

- Recommendations for dismissal.
- Giving final written warnings.
- Giving other disciplinary warnings.
- (Possibly) hearing appeals on warnings given by the Senior Receptionist.

Senior receptionist

- (Possibly) giving first written and/or verbal warnings.

The final issue to be considered in this area is *unfair dismissal*. It may be unusual for a practice manager to be complained against to an Industrial Tribunal. Nevertheless, it is valuable to understand the standards set, by law, in this area of employment practice (*see* also the section 'Ending the contract').

The law enables employers *to sack an employee fairly* for the following reasons:

- if an employee is *incapable* of doing the job; or if the employee is found not to have the required qualifications for doing the job;
- because of the employee's *misconduct* (whether gross, serious, or persistent minor misconduct);
- if the employee is redundant;
- if there is a *statutory duty or restriction* on either the employer or the employee which prevents the employment being continued;
- for *some other substantial reason* (this might cover a wide range of issues—e.g. where there is deep personal antagonism between two employees in a small work organization or where an employee commits a criminal offence outside work that makes him/her unsuitable for continued employment).

In addition, the law forbids dismissals for certain reasons which are *automatically unfair*, e.g. an employee's gender, ethnic origin, marital status, union membership, pregnancy.

If an employer wishes to dismiss an employee for one of the fair reasons (outlined above) four considerations should be taken into account.

1 The *reason* for the person's dismissal does conform with one of the statutory 'fair reasons'.
2 The employee is given a *written statement* of the reasons for his/her dismissal. Until the 1989 Employment Act, employees needed only six months' service before they acquired a legal right to a written statement of reasons for dismissal. However, now, those employed after 26 February 1990 will have to have completed two years' service before being entitled to be given such a statement.

3   The *decision* to dismiss is *reasonable* in all the circumstances of the case. (The 'circumstances' that might be taken into account are, for example, the seriousness of the actual offence, the length of service of the employee, his/her record, any mitigating factors, the size and administrative resources of the employing organization.)

4   The extent to which an employer has reasonably tried to conform to the organization's *disciplinary procedure* and the recommendations of the *ACAS Code of Practice*.

These protective rights against unfair dismissal are *not* available to all employees. Certain categories are exempt, for example:

- those who are not direct employees (e.g. independent contractors);
- employees who have *not* completed two years continuous employment with their employer on the date their contract of employment ends;
- employees who normally work less than 16 hours per week (unless they have been employed continuously for at least eight hours a week for at least five years);
- employees over the normal retiring age.

These exemptions should not imply that such employees, e.g. those with short service and part-timers, should be treated less favourably in disciplinary matters. Any employee ought to be treated according to the standards of good employment practice that are incorporated in the law. This will ensure consistency of treatment and fairness in the handling of staff.

Sick absence and ill health

This issue can often be associated with general disciplinary and dismissal matters. However, in certain cases, a different and more sensitive approach is required. ACAS, in its advisory handbook, *Discipline at Work*, draws a distinction between 'absence for reasons which may call for disciplinary action' and 'absence on grounds of illness or injury'.

Particular advice is given for this second category of absence. ACAS advice covers the following:

- the obtaining of a prognosis from the employee's GP about the likely date of his/her return to work;
- the employer's ability to require independent medical examination of the employee;
- the nature of the work that the employee might return to;
- the possibility of there being no suitable alternative employment and so the likelihood of dismissal;
- the likelihood of a person who has a long-term illness and who is unlikely to be fit enough ever to return to work, thus becoming liable to dismissal.

Finally, the ACAS handbook draws attention to 'employees with special health problems'. Particularly, it refers to alcohol or drug abuse. 'Where it is established that an employee is suffering from alcohol or drug abuse, employers should consider whether it is appropriate to treat the problem as a medical rather than a disciplinary matter. In all cases, the employee should be encouraged to seek appropriate medical assistance.'

Practice managers must remember that if they do dismiss an employee for any medical reason, they may still be required to justify their decision to dismiss if the ex-employee appeals to an Industrial Tribunal. They will have to show that their decision was 'reasonable in all the circumstances' and that they followed a fair procedure.

Varying the contract of employment

The employment relationship is, inevitably, a changing relationship. The employer may, for example, want to introduce new conditions of employment, change working practice, increase pay. Employees (possibly through their trade union) may want to claim improvements and changes. This, then, sets the scene for one final aspect of the contract of employment— *variation*.

The law relating to variation can be complex but, in the circumstances that practice managers will normally find themselves, a few straightforward words of guidance are possible for situations where change is proposed by the employer:

- make sure that employees know what the proposed change is;
- ask them if they have any views about the proposed change;
- in the light of this consultation, announce a date for the (possibly modified) change.

If the change is 'beneficial' (e.g. a pay increase or improved holiday entitlement) then most employees will consent to the change. If an employee does not actively consent to the change but tacitly accepts it (i.e. does not object) then this is generally regarded as agreement.

Difficulties can arise if any employees object to a change. Generally, courts and tribunals have supported the employer's ability to make change in the following circumstances:

- the change is in the interests of the organization's 'efficiency';
- there has been notification of the change to the employees;
- there has been consultation about the change with the employees;
- the majority of the employees have accepted the change.

Ultimately, of course, an employer can terminate existing contracts of employment (with due notice) and offer new contracts, incorporating the changed terms and conditions of employment. This, however, is not recommended as a first approach to the issue of change. It is far better, and in the interests of good staff relations, to approach change through effective communication and consultation.

Ending the contract of employment

There are several easy ways in which a contract of employment might be ended (or terminated):

- by notice to terminate from either the employer or the employee;
- by instant dismissal by the employer;
- with the expiry of a fixed-term (i.e. temporary) contract of, for example, three months or one year;
- as a result of the repudiation of the existing contract by either the employer or the employee;
- as a result of frustration (i.e. when it is difficult for the contract to be carried out).

The most common way in which contracts of employment are terminated is *by notice*. The employee gives the employer due notice (for example, one month) because he/she is taking up a job elsewhere. Or alternatively, the employer gives the employee notice to quit (because of poor performance, misconduct, redundancy, etc.).

As far as the law is concerned, the *notice to be given by the employee* is a matter for the employer to determine. Normally, this would be indicated in the initial contract of employment information and documentation. However, the *employer*, in law, is required *to give the employee certain minimum amounts of notice* depending on the individual employee's length of service (*see* Table 6.1). (As indicated in the section earlier on dismissal, these notice periods can be dispensed with if the employee's dismissal is for gross misconduct.)

Table 6.1 Period of minimum notice required from employer.

Period of employment	Notice to employee
4 weeks – 2 years	1 week
2 – 3 years	2 weeks
3 – 4 years	3 weeks
4 – 5 years	4 weeks
5 – 6 years	5 weeks
6 – 7 years	6 weeks
7 – 8 years	7 weeks
8 – 9 years	8 weeks
9 – 10 years	9 weeks
10 – 11 years	10 weeks
11 – 12 years	11 weeks
More than 12 years	12 weeks

As far as employees on *fixed-term contracts*, they should be told, initially, their date of termination. If their contract can be ended by notice *before* its expiry, then minimum notice provisions (*see* Table 6.1) will apply to such early termination.

The issue of *repudiation* of contract is complex. If a practice manager does come across a case involving this, then, it is advisable to obtain professional advice on the circumstances of the case and on the law involved.

An employer can repudiate the contract of employment by the way he treats an individual employee, e.g. by victimization, by sexual harassment, by providing a dangerous and unhealthy work environment. In such cases, the aggrieved employee may feel impelled to resign. If he/she does so, then an appeal can be made to an Industrial Tribunal alleging *'constructive dismissal'*, i.e. that the employer's behaviour was such that the employee felt forced to resign, and so this was the equivalent of dismissal.

An employee may, likewise, repudiate his/her contract of employment, for example, by failing to co-operate with the employer in the provisions of a safe working environment, by prolonged unexplained absence, by dishonesty, breach of confidentiality, etc. In such cases, the employer will institute disciplinary action against the employee. This might lead to his/her ultimate dismissal.

Frustration of contract is also a complex area. Again, if the need arises, professional advice should be obtained. It involves the situation where, as a result of some unforeseen event, it becomes difficult to carry out the contract (e.g. because of the employee's serious ill-health, imprisonment, etc.) (*see* also previous section on 'Sick absence').

If, as a practice manager, you find it necessary to sack someone, it will probably be as a result of disciplinary action. The sacking will be with or without notice. If recommended good practice is followed in these cases, then few difficulties should follow. If, however, you are faced with an Industrial Tribunal case alleging unfair dismissal, then, it is sensible to collect together the evidence and documentation that you have available and obtain professional advice about how to handle the case (*see* section on 'How employees enforce their rights').

How employees enforce their rights

There are four bodies that employees might appeal to in the first instance:

- an Industrial Tribunal;
- the County Court;
- the Equal Opportunities Commission (EOC);
- the Commission for Racial Equality (CRE).

It is most likely that an employee would, in fact, go to an Industrial Tribunal. This is widely known about. Its procedures are generally informal. It is possible for a person to be represented by a non-lawyer or by himself/herself. Despite the fact that legal aid is not available, it is a relatively cheap means of redress.

A person can go to the Industrial Tribunal to complain about the infringement of a wide range of employment rights. The entitlement to complain is often dependent on a person's length of service and the number of hours worked (see Table 6.2). Well over 80% of complaints to Industrial Tribunals relate to unfair dismissal. The next main group concerns discrimination and equal pay. A tiny proportion relate to other employment rights.

Table 6.2 Minimum qualifying periods for employment protection.

Employment protection rights	Qualifying period of continuous service Number of hours worked per week		
	Under 8 hours	Between 8 and 16 hours	16 or more hours
1 Written statement of employment terms	No right	5 years	13 weeks
2 Redundancy payment	No right	5 years	2 years
3 Guarantee payment	No right	5 years	1 month but the contract must be for at least 3 months
4 Medical suspension pay	No right	5 years	1 month
5 Maternity pay	No right	5 years at the beginning of the 11th week before confinement	2 years at the beginning of the 11th week before confinement
6 Right to return after confinement			
7 Itemized pay statement	No right	5 years	No qualifying period
8 Time off for trade union official's duties	No right	5 years	No qualifying period
9 Time off for trade union activities	No right	5 years	No qualifying period
10 Time off for public duties	No right	5 years	No qualifying period
11 Time off for redundant employee to seek work	No right	5 years	2 years
12 Time off for safety representatives	2 years	2 years	2 years
13 Time off for antenatal appointment	No qualifying period		
14 Written statement of reasons for dismissal	No right	5 years	2 years
15 Dismissal or action short of dismissal for trade union membership or activities (or non-membership)	No qualifying period		
16 Exclusion or expulsion from trade union in closed shop	No qualifying period		
17 Unfair dismissal	No right	5 years	2 years
18 Sex and race discrimination	No qualifying period		

As suggested earlier in this chapter, a practice manager should, if ever involved in an Industrial Tribunal case, take some professional advice. This could be from either a personnel officer or a lawyer competent in employment law. Despite the informality of the proceedings, issues of law are raised and discussed. There may be particular points of law, relating to the circumstances of the individual case, that the practice manager would like advice on.

It is possible for either employees or employers to go to the County Court to allege that the other party has breached the contract of employment and, consequently, sue for damages. It is extremely rare for this to happen. Again, in the unlikely event of a practice manager facing this type of legal proceedings, then she should take immediate advice from a lawyer.

The Equal Opportunities Commission and the Commission for Racial Equality will both listen to complainants. However, they only tend to take cases to an Industrial Tribunal if they believe that a new issue of principle can be tested. Both Commissions may also carry out investigations in particular organizations if they have information about patterns of discrimination that they believe need further inquiry.

The best course of action for any practice manager in relation to employment rights is to try, as far as possible, to adopt the best employment practice in relation to recruiting and handling staff. In this way, the probability of being faced with a complaint, for example to an Industrial Tribunal should be minimal.

Absence and Statutory Sick Pay

Statutory Sick Pay is a payment normally made to employees when they are away from work because of sickness. The scheme is adminstered by the employer on behalf of the State, and is commonly known as SSP. It would be useful for a practice manager to have some knowledge of the scheme in order to explain wage payments to employees.

The employer needs to do certain things even before the employee is off sick.

1 *Make sure employees know what to do if they are off sick.* It is largely up to the employers to decide how they want to be informed and when but it should be made clear to enable employees to comply.
2 *Decide if your employee is really sick.* It is usual to ask for proof in the form of either a self-certification form or a doctor's certificate. Absences of a week or less should be covered by self-certification form SC1 (which can be obtained from the DSS) or you could draft your own form. Absences of more than a week should be covered by a doctor's certificate.

3   *Make sure your employees know which days are their qualifying days.* Qualifying days are the only days of the week for which SSP has to be paid. Usually an employee's qualifying days will be the days when they are required to work under their contract with you.

SSP is paid on the fourth day of sickness absence (the first three days are known as waiting days). SSP is paid for a maximum of 28 weeks.

The current rate is (as at 6 April 1991):

Average weekly earnings	Weekly rate of SSP
£185 or more	£52.50
£52 to £184.99	£43.50

Employers should charge tax and National Insurance contributions on SSP, as though they were earnings. Employers can get back 80% of the gross SSP they have paid (this takes effect from 6 April 1991; for payments for SSP previous to this date 100% is reimburseable). They do this by taking off the amount they have paid from the amount they send to the Inland Revenue Accounts office for National Insurance contributions or PAYE income tax. Employers can also deduct an extra amount (7%) to compensate for the NI contributions they pay on SSP, this is only up to 6 April 1991.

Further guidance on how to administrate SSP is given in the following leaflets, available from the DSS:

NI 268   Employers Key: A quick guide to NI contributions/ Statutory Sick Pay
SSP 55   Tables for Statutory Sick Pay
NI 270   Employers manual on Statutory Sick Pay

Maternity leave and Statutory Maternity Pay

There are two rights concerning maternity which a practice manager should be aware of:

1   the right to return to work after maternity leave;
2   the right to maternity pay.

The first thing the practice manager would need to know before she can ascertain if either of these rights apply is the expected date of confinement. A doctor will not normally give a certificate of confinement (form MAT B1) any earlier than 14 weeks before the date of confinement so you will have to work on the date the doctor has told the employee. The practice manager will need to be kept informed if the expected date of confinement changes because she will need to recalculate as a week may make a lot of difference.

To satisfy the right to return to work ruling the employee must:

- have been continuously employed for at least 16 hours per week for a period of two years at the beginning of her 11th week before the expected week of confinement; *or*
- have been continuously employed for at least eight hours but less than 16 hours per week for a period of five years at the beginning of her 11th week before the expected week of confinement; *and*
- still be employed; *and*
- tell her employer at least 21 days before the start of the absence that she intends to return to work and the expected week of confinement.

However in the case of a company which employs five people or less at the start of the maternity leave (including the woman herself) the woman does not have the right to return to work if it is not reasonably practicable for the employer to permit her to return to work or offer her alternative employment. It is up to the employer to prove that it was not reasonably practicable in any ensuing tribunal case.

If the employee satisfies the return to work ruling she is entitled to return to a similar job which is appropriate to her qualifications and experience. It may not be precisely the same job but must not be inferior in terms of salary and conditions of employment than she would have enjoyed had she remained at work.

To satisfy the right to maternity pay ruling the employee must:

- have been continuously employed for at least 26 weeks continuing into the 15th week before her baby is due; *and*
- have average weekly earnings of not less than the lower earnings limit for the payment of National Insurance contributions; *and*
- still be pregnant at the 11th week before her expected week of confinement or have been confined by that time; *and*
- have stopped working for the employer.

Statutory Maternity Pay is payable for a maximum of 18 weeks and there are two rates of pay. The higher rate is 9/10 (90%) of the employee's average weekly earnings and is payable for the first six weeks SMP is due. For the remainder of the maternity pay period SMP is paid at the lower rate. The lower rate of SMP is a set rate which is reviewed each year and published in a leaflet NI 196. To qualify for the higher rate of SMP the employee must satisfy the following:

- have been continuously employed for at least 16 hours per week for a period of two years at the beginning of her 11th week before the expected week of confinement; *or*
- have been continuously employed for at least eight hours but less then 16 hours per week for a period of five years at the beginning of her 11th week before the expected week of confinement.

SMP paid can be recovered (including tax and usual deductions) and an extra amount to compensate for the National Insurance contributions paid on that SMP. This can be recovered by making deductions from the monthly payments of NI contributions sent to the Collector of Taxes.

For further guidance on adminstration SMP the following leaflets are very useful and are available from the DSS.

NI 257   Employers Guide to Statutory Maternity Pay

SMP 55   Tables Statutory Maternity Pay

NI 269   Employers Manual on National Insurance contributions

National Insurance

National Insurance contributions are payments made for most employees who earn more than a certain amount. Employers must make part of the payment themselves but the rest is taken from what they pay employees. There are three possible cases:

1 if the employee's earnings are below the lower earnings limit no contributions are paid by either employee or employer;
2 if the employee's earnings are above the lower earnings limit but below the upper earnings limit both the employer and the employee must pay contributions on all earnings;
3 if the employee's earnings are above the upper earnings limit your employee pays contributions on all earnings up to and including the upper earnings limit but there is no limit to the contributions paid by the employer.

The rate at which the employee's and employer's contributions are calculated depends on the earnings bracket the employee falls into.

For more details on earnings brackets and Natiional Insurance contributions see the following DSS leaflets:

NI 269   Employer's Manual on National Insurance contributions

NI 268   Employer's Key: A quick quide to National Insurance contributions/Statutory Sick Pay

To obtain any of the leaflets mentioned, contact the local DSS office or write to:
DSS Leaflets,
PO Box 21,
Stanmore,
Middlesex HA7 1AY

PAYE

PAYE stands for Pay As You Earn. It is the way most people pay their income tax. Tax is deducted from an employee's pay on a weekly or monthly basis and sent to the Inland Revenue. This saves people from having to pay all their tax in one lump sum at the end of the tax year. The tax year runs from 6 April of one year to the 5 April of the next. There are really only five main things an employer needs to do:

1 tell the tax office when a new employee starts work;
2 work out the tax due each pay day;
3 pay this to the Inland Revenue each month;
4 tell the tax office when the employee leaves;
5 tell the tax office at the end of each tax year how much each employee has earned and how much tax and National Insurance contributions have been deducted.

By contacting the tax office which already deals with the practice's business they will be able to tell practice managers which office is the PAYE tax office—it may be a different office. The PAYE tax office will give a tax reference, the name of a person to contact, and an Employer's Starter Pack which includes instructions, examples, tables and all the forms needed to operate PAYE.

7 Communication, Motivation and Teamwork

Introduction

THIS chapter consists of four parts:

- introduction;
- communication;
- motivation;
- teamwork.

Communication, motivation and teamwork are three psychological concepts, and an understanding of these is of great assistance to the practice manager. They are the essential behavioural concepts required to get the best out of people at work.

You (the practice manager) must set an example by communicating well, by being well motivated, and by working well with the doctors and with the practice staff.

Behavioural psychology

A browse through any psychology textbook reveals the fascinating world of the behavioural psychologist, and the names of the scholars who have developed analysis and theories to explain how we behave. One must however be careful, for psychologists may be misquoted; they are certainly easy to misunderstand.

You are unlikely to have much time to study behavioural psychology or the academic and theoretical basis of communication, motivation and teamwork. So a practical and action-orientated approach is taken in this chapter; a few examples are included which might encourage further study to help you to understand that most fascinating of creatures, the human being at work and play, in that most fascinating of environments, the busy general practice, where the paths of everyone in society converge.

A planned approach to get the best out of staff

To get the best out of staff, you should work to a plan. A logical sequence is:

- a programme to audit and, where necessary, to improve communication in the practice;
- a programme to assess and, where necessary, to improve the motivation of staff;

- a programme to audit and, where necessary, to improve teamwork.

Good individual work and good teamwork are the ultimate objectives, but to achieve them the practice first requires a high standard of communication and well motivated staff.

The need for training

Staff training is an essential additional requirement if staff are to be able to perform more effectively, and communicate more effectively.

Finding time for collective staff training

Many successful retail stores display a sign 'Closed until 9.30 a.m. Tuesdays for staff training'. They know that it is impossible to train staff without making special arrangements. Such training sessions for practice staff are easily laid on, without necessarily publicizing the fact to patients.

On one morning each month, one doctor and a senior receptionist can run a minimum service for patients; no appointments are booked for before 9.45 a.m. – and staff can get together from 8.30 to 9.30 a.m. for a training session. This does not take the place of other off-site training, but it does result in nine or 10 training sessions each year (it is best to omit August, December and January).

Training sessions can be led by the doctor or yourself; consider inviting someone else, for example from the local FHSA or health board if they are willing to help, or another practice manager who teaches practice management or practice reception duties. People are happy to help if asked, especially if there is a fee or a present such as a book token to reward the extra effort involved.

The need for self-audit

It should not be assumed that you will, simply by virtue of your appointment, be such a good communicator, so well motivated, such a good team leader and such a good team member that you will not need to be better trained and better motivated.

You should set aside some time on a regular basis to conduct some self-audit. Stop and think; ask youself:

- whether communication between you and the doctors is effective and harmonious?
- whether communication between you and the practice staff is equally good?
- whether you feel enthusiastic and keen about your job?
- whether you are in harmony with and in control of the practice team?

Consider discussing these matters periodically with someone in whom you are able to confide, preferably one of the doctors.

If this self-audit shows, as it may from time to time, that you need to improve your own performance in the areas of communication, motivation and teamwork, make a plan, perhaps involving some training, to improve it. Write some target dates into your plan; measure your progress and see how a planned approach can make it easier for you. If you get it right for yourself, you will find it a lot easier to get it right for the team.

Communication

In this part, the following aspects of communication will be covered: definitions, inter-personal communication, harmony-body language, clarity, listening and confirming, time and place, training staff and doctors, systems, an efficient office, practice policies and prodedures, auditing and its benefits.

Note: This part of the chapter is a carefully worked example of communication. You have not read it to the end, but already you should have a clear view of what it is about and what to expect.

What is communication?

Dictionary definitions of communication include concepts such as the transfer of information and ideas from one person to another. Everyone uses language as a written and spoken code to transfer information. Diagrams and graphs are also used as a form of code. Good communication results when the meaning of this code, this language, these diagrams, is interpreted by the receiver without error.

Body positions, facial expressions, gestures and the choice of words can change the meaning of the language, providing both a delight and a danger in human communication.

A practical approach to communication is required and in this chapter it is suggested that communication within the practice should be approached at two levels:

- inter-personal communication;
- communication systems.

Improved communication in general practice can be achieved by a variety of techniques; the more human and acceptable the technique, the more likely it is to succeed. The overriding priorities for communication in general practice are:

- efficiency;
- confidentiality.

Inter-personal communication

The aims of improving inter-personal communication are to foster harmony between individuals and to ensure efficient, secure and error-proof passage of information and ideas.

Patients quickly pick up signals, and they are quick to observe inter-personal relationships in the surgery: while waiting to see the doctor or nurse, they sit and watch receptionists, nurses and doctors coming and going; they notice any reassuring nods or cross frowns exchanged between colleagues.

Patients also hear what is said within earshot: the more interesting the subject, the more acute their hearing.

Errors in communication can be embarrassing: worse, they can be dangerous or even fatal:

'How is your mother, Mrs Smith?'
'Oh doctor, don't you know? She died last week . . . '

'We are going to repeat the smear because the laboratory found the last one difficult to interpret . . . '
'But I just heard someone saying it was abnormal . . . '

'I didn't realize that you thought it was an emergency . . . '
'Well, doctor, we just put him in the car and took him straight to hospital and he is still in intensive care . . . '

Harmony – body language

The signals sent out by body language have been analysed by behavioural psychologists. It is important not to send out the wrong signals. While there are exceptions to most rules, the following notes will, if studied, be useful in day-to-day situations.

- Upright, still, no facial expression = formal, reserved.
- Leaning forward = receptive and attentive.
- Leaning back or away = unreceptive, uninterested.
- Erect or tilted head = neutral or interested.
- Head bent down = can be judgmental or negative.
- Arms firmly folded = defensive and reserved.
- Arms relaxed, hands loosely on lap = calm and receptive.
- Ankles crossed and legs stiff = defensive and reserved.
- Legs relaxed, ankles lightly crossed = calm and receptive.
- Fidgeting or tightly clasped hands = tense.

- Eyes roaming   = tense and uncertain.
- Eyes looking at the face of the   = confident and interested.
  other person
- Hands still, open palms outward   = confident and relaxed.
- Fingers clenched   = tense.
- Leaning back in the chair, hands   = I know it all.
  locked behind the head (male)
- Leaning back in the chair, hands   = look at me.
  locked behind the head (female)

If you sometimes feel embarrassed or awkward in particular situations, analyse why and see if you can do something about it.

- Get the positions of tables, desks and chairs right – too close intrudes on personal ease; across the desk can be confrontational; low easy chairs can make women in short skirts feel awkward.
- If two or three of you are working on a paper, consider sitting between or to the side of one another on one side of a table, and working together on one copy.
- Consider having some paper and a pencil handy to draw a diagram, or to make notes to break up the stiffness.
- Above all, think about it and do not be shy of discussing such difficulties with colleagues: few of us will not admit to feeling awkward sometimes and we can best learn to overcome this by sharing the problem and learning from others.

Improving personal communication – clarity

Errors and misunderstandings in communication can be avoided by:

- thinking carefully in advance about what it is you wish to communicate and making notes if approriate;
- keeping your message clear and simple;
- not hiding your message in a mass of detail.

A useful technique is to make notes under these three headings:

- *Must* – what is essential?
- *Should* – what, if not mentioned, could cause problems?
- *Could* – there is a lot one *could* say . . . but unless it is a *must* or a *should*, leave it out.

It is essential to get straight to the point, unless it is clearly appropriate to have a chat to relax the atmosphere and then steer the conversation on to the essentials.

If you say, 'I am 'phoning to ask if you could act as locum next weekend', the doctor at the other end gets the point at once. Starting the conversation with along explanation of the difficulties in meeting various commitments at this time of the year does not necessarily soften the doctor up and make him more likely to say yes – it is more likely to confuse and irritate him.

Listening and confirming

Communication is more than putting it across to others. It is, of course, a two-way process. It is essential that you ensure that *you understand them* and that *they understand you.*

You can learn from taxi drivers who usually repeat the name and address of the next call to the radio controller so that there is no possibility of misunderstanding and error; aircraft pilots have similar drills.

On important matters, and always if patients are upset or if their first language is not English, you must spend some time confirming so that there is no room for confusion.

Time and place

You will know how you feel when several people stop you in the corridor when you are in a hurry and raise important matters; and how often you forget something when you are not given a chance to attend to it at the right place and the right time.

It is important to think not only of your own time and pressures, but also those of others. Thinking about the right moment and the right place is an important part of good communication.

You should insist that raising important matters casually is unacceptable. You should insist on a note to confirm an oral request being written by the person concerned; and insist that there should be a proper discussion at an appropriate time.

Training staff

Appropriate training invariably improves performance. Time spent training staff in communication skills and techniques, and in discussing communication with practice staff, is rarely wasted. Everyone can produce an anecdote from personal or working experience about how communication broke down. You should keep inter-personal skills in mind when identifying individual and collective training needs.

Training doctors

One hopes that most practice managers will find that the communication skills of newly trained doctors are well developed; but it cannot be assumed that newly arrived doctors know all the unwritten rules and customs of a practice. Written guidance and practice procedures are essential to good communication. A series of procedure notes can be built up over time, kept up to date, and given to all new arrivals so that they know how the routine of the practice runs. These are described more fully later (*see* page 90).

Doctors are subject to as many stresses and strains as the rest of us and their communication skills may suffer under pressure. If there are any problems in communication between doctors and others, you must not be shy of analysing the problem and finding a proper, tactful and productive solution. If it is not easy to mention the matter to the doctor concerned, it may be preferable to involve doctors in discussions about communication difficulties and to organize inter-personal communication training and involve the doctors.

Communication systems

The essential principles of communication systems in general practice are:

- communication is a matter for everyone in the practice;
- communication requires systematic thought and study;
- communication can be improved by audit and training;
- the interests of patients, doctors and indeed all staff must be uppermost in everyone's mind, particularly in regard to confidentiality.

Communication systems include:

- written communications sent to people such as letters, memoranda;
- notice boards;
- medical records;
- message books, day books, desk diaries and hand over books;
- routine and special practice meetings.

The main dangers are:

- that paper does not reach the person or is seen by the wrong person;
- that doctors or staff are on leave when a notice appears;
- that there is no system to brief those absent from meetings.

An efficient office

In a well organized office, communication should rarely be a problem. One well known practice, which has new premises designed to ensure good communication, and whose former manager is an authority on practice management, uses the following techniques.

- Each doctor has an 'in-basket' with the doctor's name on it; all incoming mail is put into it (the usual procedure in most practices).
- Each doctor has a separate knee hole work space in a large shared office to do administrative work. Doctors see patients in the consulting room, and do other work in this office; there is rarely more than one doctor there at any one time. When there doing administrative work, doctors are near the staff for ease of communication.
- Any letter to be seen by all the doctors is photocopied and put into all the 'in-baskets' in this central administrative office within minutes of receipt. This is easily done as the photocopying machine, doctor's administrative office and staff are within a few steps.
- All practice meetings are minuted, a copy of the minutes going into all the 'in-baskets', thereby covering the problem of the absent doctor and the doctor called out of the meeting to attend to an emergency.
- In the adminstrative office, there are three white notice boards on the wall (coloured felt tip pens are used), visible to doctors and nurses as they come and go throughout the day and throughout the week. About three weeks' information is retained – starting again at the top and rubbing out a week at a time.
- One notice board is for birth/deaths, one for hospital admissions/discharges, and one for important notes about patients (e.g. house fire, invalid relative staying for a week).

You should work out what systems are required to maintain and improve communication. Discussion with other practice managers and the occasional visit to another practice can stimulate good new ideas.

Practice policies and procedures

You should have, in writing, a set of practice policies and procedures. These form part of the management of the practice routine but are also examples of communication systems. The following examples indicate the some of the subjects which need to be covered:

- calendar of public holidays and doctors'/staff holidays;
- how to submit leave requests;
- procedure for notifying sickness absence;
- programme of visitors to the practice.

Auditing communication in the practice

It is not essential to try to audit the quality of communication in the practice, but it can be a really useful exercise, especially if you do it on a systematic basis. A simple and practical way of doing this is to design a questionnaire, and get the doctors and the practice staff to complete it. Depending on how well established the working relationships are, the questionnaires can be anonymous or have names on them.

Suitable questions will vary as practices are so different, but Fig. 7.1 shows an example of how you might approach the task of designing a simple questionnaire to test the quality of communication.

Dear Colleague,

Practice Communications Audit

As agreed at the recent practice meeting, I am writing to ask for your help with a short check on how effective communication is in the practice. Please complete the attached questionnaire and put it in my internal mail tray. As it is a first attempt, I am making the questionnaire anonymous so that no one need worry about what they put down. The results will be published on the staff notice board and discussed at the next meeting of staff and doctors on (date). Many thanks.

(signed)

Practice Manager.

Communications systems in the practice

(please write the answer number in the brackets)

5 = excellent
4 = satisfactory
3 = adequate but improvement needed
2 = inadequate, major improvements needed
1 = poor, a real problem

Do you feel that there is a well-understood method of informing doctors about incoming 'phone calls?   ( )

Are our methods of getting information to staff, especially part-timers, reliable?   ( )

Do you know well enough in advance, and as far as the practice is concerned, when you will be able to take annual leave?   ( )

Do you find out about what is going on in the practice in a reliable way in which you have confidence?   ( )

What do you think of the system for fire precautions?   ( )

Inter-personal communications

Do you feel that it is easy to let the doctors/staff know if you have problems contacting them?   ( )

Do you feel that the doctors/staff appreciate the difficulties involved in fitting in urgent consultations when surgeries are already fully booked?   ( )

How would you rate your understanding of the doctors'/staff's greatest difficulties with administration? (this is an example of an obscure question – reword it and avoid obscure questions!)   ( )

Figure 7.1 Practice communications audit.

The benefits of a regular audit of communication

These include:

- putting the matter on everyone's agenda and getting them thinking about it;
- providing the stimulus to everyone to discuss communication problems informally and then at a meeting;
- letting the doctors know if their staff have problems communicating with them and with patients;
- providing the opportunity to compare the results of audits; the same questions can be used again periodically in a cycle and the improving (or deteriorating!) results put on the notice board.

There may be someone in the practice who is particularly interested in questionnaires: do not hesitate to ask others to work on the questionnaire with you, or to produce the questions.

If every staff group (the doctors, the receptionists, the secretaries) gets a turn to set the questions, you will find that they ask questions designed to test the areas of communication which they think need improvement. Activities such as this foster good communication, help to motivate staff by involving them in checking how communications are working, and are useful in team building.

Motivation

Before reading further, you might find it helpful to glance ahead at the headings in the part of the section about motivation; this will give you a feel for the topic before you go any further. Before doing so, be assured that the rather grand sounding sections about behavioural psychology and Maslow's theory are very straightforward.

What is motivation?

Motivation is that human instinct, feeling, or emotion, that impels or drives us into action; it puts energy and direction into our behaviour; it incites the will.

The concept of motivation includes:

- needs, driving forces;
- motives, reasons for working well, goals;
- personal ambitions and expectations;
- encouragement, stimulus;
- inducement, reward.

Assessing motivation

The extent to which staff are well motivated is not easy to audit or measure. It is largely a matter of assessing staff morale, willingness to co-operate and personal attitudes.

The assessment of morale and motivation is usually best done subjectively by the doctors and the practice manager and discussed at that level. Staff motivation should be reviewed and discussed at least annually, usually before decisions are made about the next year's pay levels. Reviews can be more frequent if the doctors and the practice manager become aware that the staff are less content than usual, or if there are unexpected staff resignations.

Ways of motivating staff

The usual ways of motivating staff are:

- involving them in achieving the objectives of the organization;
- furthering their personal development and training; giving them increased responsibility whenever possible;
- giving them appropriate praise, rewards and benefits;
- making the workplace pleasant, having a cheerful atmosphere and fun at work when appropriate; and fostering social relationships between colleagues.

Techniques used to motivate people have the following factors in common:

- helping them to appreciate, more fully, the importance of the organization for which they are working:
- helping them to realize the importance of their personal contribution to the aims of the organization;
- helping them to enjoy their work and contribute even more;
- giving them clearly defined areas of work and giving them recognition for their achievements;
- rewarding them both materially and emotionally for improving their contribution.

Maslow's theory of human motivation

The American behavioural psychologist, Abraham Harold Maslow (1908–1970) described a hierarchy of seven human needs.

1 Physiological needs: food, water, temperature control.
2 Safety needs: security, freedom from threat.

3 Social needs: love, affiliation, acceptance by others.
4 Esteem needs: both self-esteem and esteem from others, prestige, status.
5 Cognitive needs: knowledge, understanding, curiosity.
6 Aesthetic needs: order, beauty, structure, art.
7 Self-fulfilment needs: achievement, realization of potential.

Maslow's theory of human motivation depends on the seven needs being a hierarchy; unless there is a hierarchical relationship between the seven needs, i.e. unless they must come in that sequence and have a rank value, all you have is a list which you can put in any sequence. To Maslow, a starving person was, for example, unlikely to be much concerned with self-esteem.

If you accept Maslow's theory, its significance for you as a practice manager is that it provides a useful list of factors affecting motivation; the hierarchy or ranking theory is useful to the extent that one must get the basics right first before expecting more of staff. However, it is unwise to use it too rigidly: for example, although Maslow ranks aesthetic needs above self-fulfilment needs, in the working situation self-fulfilment needs are probably more important than aesthetic needs.

The Maslow needs can be met in the working situation: think about and add to these brief examples:

Maslow's hierarchy number	Example
1	Good catering arrangements
2	Secure conditions of employment, contracts, job descriptions, fairness
3	Social functions
4	Praise for good work. Name/job title badges
5	Training and learning opportunities
6	Attractive environment, orderly systems, flowers, good background music
7	Identification of training needs, encouragement for staff to develop their careers, skills and knowledge.

Performance appraisal

Performance appraisal is a modern personnel management technique intended to help to motivate people. It codifies an age old process of working out 'How well are they doing?' There is nothing new and gimmicky about performance appraisal other than its name and some of the associated jargon.

If used well, a performance appraisal scheme can be popular and of substantial benefit in a practice. It must however be used only after careful preparation and with an understanding of what can go wrong if it is not used properly.

The aims of performance appraisal

- To motivate staff.
- To enable them to be clear about the job performance expected of them.
- To enable them to learn in a methodical and consistent way how the practice manager considers they are performing, and to discuss training needs.
- To help them to understand more completely how their work affects, and inter-relates with, the work of others.
- To provide them with a regular opportunity to raise issues with the practice manager which might not otherwise be raised on a day-to-day basis.

A performance appraisal system consists of:

- the setting of objectives;
- planned personal development;
- monitoring;
- assessment.

The performance appraisal process

The performance appraisal process usually consists of four components:

- setting objectives;
- having periodic monitoring meetings (e.g. monthly, quarterly);
- having periodic appraisal meetings; normally annually but for newly employed staff or staff with particular difficulties, perhaps twice a year or even more;
- having the results of appraisal reviewed.

Introducing and running a performance appraisal system

The components of the introduction and conduct of a performance appraisal system include:

- planning the system;
- obtaining the consent of the doctors;
- introducing the concept to the existing staff;
- agreeing objectives with each member of the staff;

- drawing up the timetable;
- setting up the paperwork and confidential filing system;
- drawing up a monitoring and performance appraisal programme for the next 18 months, reviewing it and updating it every six months; and adhering to it;
- having regular monitoring meetings;
- conducting periodic performance appraisal meetings;
- conducting the review process;
- reviewing and modifying objectives as time passes, as staff develop, as individuals leave and join the staff, and as practice circumstances change.

Voluntary or compulsory?

It is usual, when introducing a performance appraisal scheme, to make it voluntary for existing employees and compulsory only for new employees. No matter how useful, modern techniques do not invariably find favour, particularly with those who are either exceptionally competent and who might scorn the technique, or who lack self-confidence and who might find the technique threatening.

It is possible to make performance appraisal voluntary even for new employees, in which case a salary lead may be given to those who accept it.

Exclusions – appraisal of whom?

Performance appraisal and objective setting are appropriate for the more senior staff: while cleaners should have their punctuality and the quality of their work supervised, any slackness checked and their good work acknowledged and praised, formal appraisal schemes are inappropriate for them. It would be difficult to set objectives for cleaners and involve them in the objective setting process. Although this is a matter of opinion, a short task list and an occasional informal discussion about work is usually more appropriate than a performance appraisal scheme for staff in posts with uncomplicated clerical or manual duties.

Deciding whether to introduce performance appraisal

The factors which should to be taken into account when deciding whether to introduce a performance appraisal scheme include positive, negative and neutral factors.

Positive factors are factors leading to a decision to introduce a performance appraisal scheme which will:

- improve performance if used well;
- avoid the feeling that no one ever bothers to consider how people work;

- provide the opportunity to praise good work and help staff, by identifying and planning any training needed, and by tactfully giving any advice needed to improve performance;
- provide the practice manager with a structure for counselling, disciplining and if unavoidable having the doctors dismiss any member of staff who does not work at an acceptable level of attendance and performance despite appraisal, counselling and disciplinary warnings.

Negative factors are factors leading to a decision not to introduce an appraisal scheme because it may:

- cause suspicion and anxiety among existing staff;
- damage, or even be counter-productive if not used well or if staff were to rebel against it;
- requires too much time for preparation and implementation.

Other factors are factors which should be considered before deciding to introduce performance appraisal.

- If job descriptions are up to date, staff in post are happy and properly paid, and there is a feeling of mutual confidence between doctors, the practice manager and the staff, a performance appraisal system is easier to operate and more likely to succeed.
- It involves a significant use of resources and a degree of risk. It therefore must be approved by all the doctors in the practice.
- It requires a skilled and confident practice manager if it is to succeed.
- It is difficult to determine in advance whether it will be cost-effective.
- It is usually only suitable in very large practices.

Consistency and fairness

Consistency and fairness are normally achieved by having three participants: the post-holder, the appraiser (the practice manager), and the reviewer (a doctor).

How confidential is the process?

In theory the entire process including the fact that someone is being appraised, where the performance appraisal is to take place, and the results of the performance appraisal, should be confidential to the three participants.

Most of the completed documentation is confidential to the member of staff, the appraiser and the reviewer. It is possible for certain documents to be made generally available: for example if the practice manager is the subject of performance appraisal, it is very useful for the other employees to see the objectives of the practice manager; and it is best for everyone involved to agree at the outset to have their objectives circulated to everyone else in the team.

Performance appraisal meetings

In order to avoid trouble and tension, appraisal meetings must:

- contain no surprises; any adverse comment should already have been made at earlier monitoring and counselling meetings;
- be discussed by the practice manager and a doctor if the performance of the individual is below par and if the interview is likely to cause any upset;
- be prepared for with the greatest care by the practice manager;
- be conducted in privacy, without interruption, and in comfortable and non-threatening surroundings;
- be conducted on the basis of 'do as you would be done by'. The appraiser must first, while preparing, think how the appraisal meeting will appear to the member of staff, and conduct the meeting with the greatest sensitivity for the feelings and aspirations of the other person;
- be part of the motivation process.

Format of a performance appraisal meeting

While there is no mandatory format, it is useful if the appraiser has a short preliminary meeting with the post-holder, to explain where the meeting will be held, when, and the general format. It is preferable to try to find somewhere away from the practice, or to choose a time when there are few people around and no likelihood of interruption. It helps if the post-holder is told something along these lines:

'I'd like to give you an idea of how I'd like to cover the ground at our performance appraisal meeting. I've made some notes for you and I'll give you them in a minute; so there is no need to write anything down just now.

We will start by looking at the objectives we agreed for you for the year. I'd like to discuss how realistic they were, what happened in terms of resource restrictions, and any unexpected new priorities that made if difficult for you to achieve any of the objectives, and what we have both learned about objective setting in the light of this first year of the process.

Then I'd like to go over each one, so that we can discuss what went well and what you would have liked to improve on. This should lead us on to discussing your training needs for the next year or 18 months.

Then over to you, your chance to raise anything you want to discuss. Don't be shy because this is your chance to say anything you want to say in confidence.

There is no need to feel nervous. If there has been anything that has needed attention during the year, it will already have been mentioned. So there will be no surprises.

It is important that at the end of the meeting you feel that you have been given a really fair chance to look at the past year and the next year with me. If you go home feeling confident, and if you start the next day feeling that you want to go at it even harder, and even more happily, then we will have succeeded.'

Review process

The results of the performance appraisal should be recorded on simple suitably designed forms reproduced in the practice, and filed securely. To ensure consistency and fairness, the process should be reviewed by someone next in line up from the appraiser. In a practice, the practice manager will normally do all the staff performance appraisals, and a doctor will normally be the person who does the reviewing.

At the outset, you should secure the genuine and interested co-operation and assistance of at least one doctor in the practice, with whom the entire process should be discussed. There is no set format for a review process, but normally the appraiser should discuss the performance appraisal meeting in advance with the reviewer, then report back after it has been completed; it is a matter of opinion whether the post-holder should have the review conducted in a group of three, or whether the post-holder should see the reviewer separately and alone.

Finally, please note that throughout this section, the word 'meeting' has been used for performance appraisal and review, and not the word 'interview'. This is deliberate, and important; it is essential to have a meeting of minds and not an interviewer/interviewee situation at the sensitive time of performance appraisal.

Timing

Most practices have a time of the year at which the question of salary increases for staff is discussed. This is usually a tense time and staff are usually glad when the uncertainty is over and matters are decided. It is unwise to mix salary discussions with performance appraisal.

Objective setting

The appraisal process is critically dependent on the setting of objectives. The setting of objectives is a technique which requires knowledge and skill; it can be greatly improved by training. If objectives are not accurate and relevant, the performance appraisal process becomes difficult. Unrealistic or vaguely described objectives are quickly recognized as such by the member of staff and they will rapidly discredit the appraisal process.

Objectives must be:

- comprehensive (covering the range of duties);
- achievable (adequately resourced in terms of time, money and knowledge);
- measurable (in terms of time and extent of achievement);
- fair (e.g. not expecting too advanced a quality of work from those without adequate knowledge and experience; achievable within the working hours of the individual).

There should normally not be less than six and no more than eight objectives set for each individual. Each objective must in itself be a critical success factor: if all are achieved, the job will have been successfully done. Each objective should be clearly and comprehensively described: who must do what, by when and within what limits. The aim or outcome of success should also be defined.

The following examples of vague objectives for a practice manager will help readers to understand the difficulties in setting objectives.

1   To make the routine of the practice run better (better than what?).
2   To get staff to work better (better than what?).
3   To avoid waste of money (how is waste of money measured?).
4   To avoid waste of time (how is waste of time measured?).

You could have, as objectives, the following seven key tasks:

- to establish a practice training policy and to have it agreed by the doctors and the staff within four months;
- to organize a business planning seminar for the doctors, the practice manager and the practice accountant, within 12 months, the aim of the seminar being to define the practice objectives, to cost them, and to agree a programme to achieve them and measure progress and cost outturn;
- in discussion with staff, to determine the training needs of every individual for the next two years, and to discuss staff training needs with the doctors within six months;
- within a budget of one week's net salary per head, to ensure that every member of staff who wishes to benefit from training attends a training course which meets identified training needs, within 15 months;
- to convert the medical record envelope system to an A4 folder system within 12 months for an expenditure of not more than x pence per record;
- in co-operation with the practice accountant, and within six months, to identify achievable savings in practice expenditure so that the gross income to net income ratio of the partners might be improved by a target amount of 5%, and so that the costs of staff training can be met without reduction in net income to the partners;
- to introduce performance appraisal for the three senior receptionists within eight months;

- to conduct two patient satisfaction surveys within 12 months with the aim of identifying changes to practice routine and practice procedures which will improve the patients' perception of the practice as a caring and responsive organization.

A practice manager with such a list of objectives would have to make a plan for achieving them, making allowances for personal annual leave, doctors' annual leave, avoiding the difficult periods of Easter, Christmas and the New Year, and times such as school half-term holidays.

Soon, the available periods of time in the year for working on such objectives would become clear; activity would be focused; and instead of going to work every Monday with the intention of 'getting things done' and going home at the end of the week with that frustrating feeling of having been driven by events and not having achieved enough, there is a chance that the practice manager will have had to put a 'do not disturb' notice on the door from time to time to complete certain tasks by identified deadlines.

At the end of four to six months with the above objectives, a practice manager might, in reviewing achievements, note and report to the doctors:

- the practice training policy had been agreed on time;
- the business planning seminar could not be achieved within existing constraints of time and knowledge within the practice, but that it could be 'bought in' by attendance at a training course on service management and business planning during the weekend of . . . at an estimated cost of . . . ;
- a start had been made on the conversion of records. Within the budget allocated the exercise is likely to be completed within 15 months of starting. With a temporary increase in staff hours of x hours per week (for which the FHSA or health board seems likely to reimburse 70%), the exercise could be completed in 10 months from starting, thereby reducing non-availability of records and improving efficiency and service to both patients and doctors; provided a decision is made and acted on by (date);
- the initial part of the survey of expenses (capital expenditure policy) indicated that by replacing the existing cars on the planned programme with smaller diesel-engined cars, a saving of £x per annum could be achieved (£y if smaller turbo-diesels were purchased);
- two of the three senior receptionists have agreed to performance appraisal, have attended a one-day course about it organized by the local health authority for their own staff, and objective setting is in progress. (The third senior receptionist having given a week's notice on the grounds that performance appraisal is the 'thin end of the wedge');
- it will be possible to conduct only one patient-satisfaction survey with existing resources.

In other words, objectives will not easily be achieved within the contraints of time and other resources without some upset. Inability to achieve objectives because of lack of resources or other valid reasons does not constitute failure on the part of the individual – a point which *must* be stressed when discussing the introduction of a performance appraisal system, and constantly repeated if staff feel threatened.

Personal development and training

The identification of training needs is a key part of the performance appraisal process. A practice should have a training and development policy: otherwise training needs, once identified, may be left unmet, causing the staff to wonder why so much trouble has been taken to identify training needs when no opportunities for training are provided.

A policy for training and development is a rather grandiose phrase; which means in this context that doctors must agree with the practice manager that staff will have access to training and that, if necessary, staff will cover for absent colleagues, and travel costs and fees for training will, if not met from external sources, be paid for by the practice.

A training policy should include factors such as:

- the identification of the staff eligible;
- the type and location of training;
- the annual and quarterly budget provision;
- how staff should go about identifying their training needs and asking for training.

The policy need not be too detailed and specific: everyone concerned – doctors, the practice manager and the staff can be relied upon to act wisely and to seek and attend training which is known to be worthwhile.

An example of training policy.

1   All members of the management and administrative staff are expected to consider what training would improve their job performance. Training is not an entitlement, but staff should seek consent to attend at least one training course each year.
2   Training courses should be local if possible and organized by an established training institution.
3   Training should be relevant to present or expected future work in the practice.
4   The identification of training needs is the joint responsibility of the practice manager and individual members of staff; it will be on the agenda at every performance appraisal meeting.

Teamwork

What is teamwork?

Teamwork is defined in one dictionary as 'work performed by several persons in collaboration; the ability of a group to collaborate harmoniously'.

Ten people working as a team should be able to produce a higher standard of work than 10 people working individually. They should be capable of doing difficult work which 10 people working individually could not do; and doing more work than 10 people could do individually.

Primary and secondary groups

Many behavioural psychologists seem to have shied away from the team as a subject for study; most relevant work is about groups. They describe primary groups, such as families; and secondary groups, where the common purpose which is identified as essential to a group, exists in only one part of an individual's life or activity.

To behavioural psychologists, general practice teams are secondary groups; and teamwork is 'group dynamics', in which components within the group such as power, power shifts, leadership, group formation, cohesiveness, co-operation and decision-making are studied. Some consider that these components only emerge when a group or social unit is small enough for significant interactions between its members.

Motivation and team balance

What relevance does this have for the practice manager? There are three main conclusions to draw. It is essential:

- to build up and maintain a good team and think about what motivates people when selecting staff;
- to select a balance of types of people to make up a good team;
- to manage and co-ordinate their efforts in such a way as to produce the benefits which teamwork offers, which a collection of individuals cannot offer.

The first conclusion about assessing human motivation at the selection stage, can be explained thus: for some of you, your primary group or family is your main motivating influence, with the result that a job is little more than a source of variety and extra income. You may have little ambition and little driving force or motivation for promotion or progress at work: your energies are mainly devoted to your families. You find that most of your 'Maslow needs' are adequately fulfilled at home. It may not be easy or even possible to motivate you to become very involved at work.

For others, your 'Maslow needs' are not adequately fulfilled in a primary group or family. You may find that no matter how much you put into caring for your loved ones and your homes, you still require a secondary group in which to obtain further fulfilment. There are many who choose to make their work their primary group and for whom it is their main motivating interest in life.

The second conclusion is that in selecting members of the team you need to look hard at what you require. Some jobs, like cleaners or typists, need the steady worker without a great deal of ambition. Others, for example the computerizing of the records of the practice, require an imaginative and progressive person who is always looking for opportunities in systems, who is ambitious for the outcome of the work and also personally ambitious. Such people are more easily motivated in the secondary group or practice team.

The third conclusion is that the practice manager must, in planning and developing the structure of the practice and the team, put together complementary job descriptions. This is to build up sub-groups, each with their own built-in leadership, to whom tasks can be delegated, and in which loyalty and standards of excellence can be fostered. This is usually done by having one senior receptionist and one senior secretary and so on. If they are given areas of responsibility, the practice manager's leadership task is shared, individual creativity is released, and morale and performance are improved.

What is a primary health care team?

An accepted definition, written before the need for practice managers became apparent, is:

> 'A primary health care team is an interdependent group of general medical practitioners, secretaries, receptionists and practice nurses who, together with health visitors, community nurses and midwives, share a common purpose and responsibility, each member clearly understanding their functions and those of other members, so that they all pool skills and knowledge to provide an effective primary health care service.'

It is essential to distinguish the clinical management roles of professionally qualified staff, which usually form no part of the practice manager's role, from the practice business and administrative responsibilities which do. There are, of course exceptions if the practice manager is one of the doctors, or a nurse who also has clinical management and co-ordination duties.

Team member selection

In selecting the team, you need a balance; if everyone is a steady worker with no development potential, progress will be slow. If everyone is imaginative and ambitious, the basic work may suffer. It is the practice manager's job to achieve a balance, and through wise selection, to build a balanced and competent team.

Team building

Team building depends on establishing mutual trust and confidence among the people around you. You must be good at your job and people must trust you and find you easy to get on with if you are to have a good team.

Essentials of teamwork

It is useful to put down on paper your own list of the essentials of teamwork in your practice; and in a seminar or group work to ask the various members of the practice staff to contribute their ideas about what teamwork means to them. The exercise of defining teamwork in a group is valuable in helping staff to think and work as a team.

A list of components could look like this:

- work performed by several persons;
- ability of a group to collaborate harmoniously;
- ability of a group to work together effectively;
- group work co-ordinated by a leader;
- work for patients by persons with complementary skills;
- work to high standards of care and confidentiality;
- combined and effective effort.

There are useful words in building up the concept of a team in group work, e.g. team, group, faction, clique, co-operation, collaboration, esprit de corps, harmony. If staff are provided with or asked to bring dictionaries and even a thesaurus or two for a team-building session, they can produce many such words without feeling tongue-tied or less well educated than others.

It is usually productive to get staff working in small groups first to suggest the words that occur to them; and then with everyone together by asking for their concepts; putting concepts to them to approve or disapprove (team and group being examples of good ones, faction and clique being examples of bad ones) can be entertaining.

If staff build up their local concept of what a good team should be, and what kind of team they like, they develop a feeling that they are making the rules for themselves rather than having them imposed (i.e. 'ownership of the team concept').

The effective team

In *How To Be An Even Better Manager* Michael Armstrong quotes the following description of the main features of an effective team.

1   The atmosphere tends to be informal, comfortable, relaxed.
2   There is a lot of discussion in which initially everyone participates, but it remains pertinent to the task of the group.
3   The task or objective of the group is well understood and accepted by the members. There will have been free discussion of the objectives at some point until it was formulated in such a way as the members of the group would commit themselves to it.
4   The members listen to each other. Every idea is given a hearing. People do not appear to be afraid of putting forward a creative thought, even if it seems fairly extreme.
5   There is disagreement. Disagreements are not suppressed or over-ridden by premature group action. The reasons are carefully examined, and the group seeks to resolve them rather than to dominate the dissenter.
6   Most decisions are reached by a kind of consensus in which it is clear that everybody is in general agreement and willing to go along.
7   Criticism is frequent, frank and relatively comfortable. There is little evidence of personal attack, either openly or in a hidden fashion.
8   People are free in expressing their feelings as well as their ideas both on the problem and on the group's operation.
9   When action is taken, clear assignments are made and accepted.
10 The leader of the group does not dominate it, nor does the group defer unduly to the leader.'

Stages in developing a team

The four clearly definable stages in developing a team are illustrated in Fig. 7.2 (*see* page 107).

Auditing teamwork

While not essential, it can be useful to audit the quality of teamwork from time to time. At first, or if there are signs that the team is not performing well together, a questionnaire approach can be hazardous. Subjective assessment with the doctors and some development work and training can be a preferable technique in the beginning.

Once you have some confidence that teamwork is improving or after a seminar or group session to develop the concept of the team along the lines described earlier, a questionnaire can be used. There is no standard

Stage 1
Undeveloped team

Feelings not dealt with. Workplace is for work. Established line prevails. Not 'rocking the boat'. Poor listening. Weakneses covered up. Unclear objectives. Low involvement in planning. Bureaucracy. Boss takes most decisions.

Stage 2
Experimenting team

Experimentation. Risky issues debated. Wider options considered. Personal feelings raised. More listening. Concern for others.

Stage 3
Consolidating team

Experimentation. Risky issues debated. Wider options considered. Personal feelings raised. More listening. Concern for others. Methodical working. Agreed procedures. Established ground rules.

Stage 4
Mature team

Experimentation. Risky issues debated. Wider options considered. Personal feelings raised. More listening. Concern for others. Methodical working. Agreed procedures. Established ground rules. High flexibility. Appropriate leadership. Maximum use of energy and ability. Essential principles and social aspects considered. Needs of all met. Development a priority.

Figure 7.2   The four stages of team development.

approach to this, and you could usefully get each sub-group of staff to work with you to sign the questions to be asked of all members of the team, including of course the doctors. The doctors could be asked to design a questionnaire, thus giving everyone the chance to get their concerns and ideas about how the team is performing onto the agenda.

An alternative is to use the 'suggestion box' technique. After discussing the idea at a practice meeting, ask everyone in the practice to write down five weaknesses in the way the team operates, and five suggestions for improving matters. Unlike the permanent suggestion box, which is usually used intensively at first and then forgotten, fixing a time limit and then holding a training session to review perceived weaknesses and helpful suggestions is effective; it is part of teamwork and part of keeping the team working well together.

Social fucntions

Finally, do not forget the importance of the occasional social function. It can be difficult to find a suitable date, but an office party, bringing together doctors, staff and their partners is usually very popular, not particularly expensive, and worth as much as a good training session or seminar. It is also a lot more fun!

Conclusion

Throughout this chapter, the connections and inter-relationships between communication, motivation and teamwork will have become increasingly apparent:

- good communication makes good teamwork easier;
- good teamwork makes good communication easier;
- good motivation encourages good teamwork and good communication;
- good teamwork and good communication make motivation easier.

You will find that once these three psychological concepts are understood, and the team becomes increasingly familiar with them, and gradually senses the improvements they bring, there will be a snowball effect. Provided staff are well managed in these three areas by the doctors and the practice manager working in harmony, the improvement becomes cumulative. Life at work becomes more and more successful for everyone involved, going to work becomes more and more of a pleasure, and the days slip by with a greater sense of fulfilment.

Get started on the logical sequence, that plan to improve communications, motivation and teamwork with which this chapter started. Try it – it works! Good luck!

8   Health and Safety in the Surgery

THE duties of an employer arising from the Health and Safety at Work Act 1974 are not difficult to understand or to apply. Most surgery premises should meet the Act's requirements and its regulations; apart from some minor technical matters there is little in the legislation that should worry a GP.

Surgery premises are included in the 'health services' grouping and they are inspected by an official of the Health and Safety Executive (HSE) and not, as often assumed, by a local government environmental officer. HSE inspectors visit GP surgeries from time to time, and the frequency of these visits is increasing. This section of the book provides guidance on those matters which an HSE inspector may discuss with the practice manager and her staff. It does not provide a definitive statement or interpretation of the legislation.

The legislation requires an employer, including a self-employed person, to provide and maintain a safe working environment. The Act has established powers and penalties to enforce safety laws. Like most employment legislation, this law pays little regard to the limited resources of a small employer. Many of its provisions are aimed at companies where trade unions are recognized. For instance, the law states that union safety representatives and safety committees should be appointed if these are requested by a recognized union. However, even a GP who employs only a handful of staff with no union members has important duties under this Act.

The employer's duties to his staff

The main aim of the Act is to make both employers and employees conscious of the need for safety in all aspects of the day-to-day working environment. The most important duties are those which any employer must fulfil to his staff:

> '*It shall be the duty of every employer to ensure, so far as is reasonably practicable, the health, safety and welfare at work of all his employees.*'
> Health and Safety at Work Act, 1974.

Thus every employer must do all is *reasonably practicable* to ensure the well-being of his employees.

What does reasonably practicable mean?

The meaning of 'reasonably practicable' can be drawn from case law and the advice of HSE inspectors. Any proceedings taken under the Act are criminal and any employee can report to the HSE a breach of an employer's statutory duty. The HSE may then bring criminal charges.

A court's assessment of whether it was 'reasonably practicable' to avoid a particular hazard or risk of injury takes account of the cost of preventative action (particularly if the employer has few staff and limited resources) and weighs this against the risk of injury and its possible severity. Thus in general practice, a larger practice would carry a heavier burden of responsibility than one with fewer staff and resources.

Box 8.1: The Health and Safety at Work Act, 1974

The Act requires equipment and methods of working to be safe and without risk to health. Attention should be paid to waste-bins, electric typewriters, sterilizers, photocopying machines, heating equipment, computing, furniture, fire extinguishers, electrical plugs and points, light switches, and any other equipment that may be hazardous. The maintenance and renewal of equipment is particularly important. HSE inspectors look at arrangements for regular servicing, e.g. maintenance contracts for typewriters, servicing contracts for fire extinguishers, and also the age, reliability and positioning of equipment.

It is not enough to ensure that equipment and methods of working are safe. Safe systems of working need to be understood by all staff and applied.

Written statement of safety policy

The law requires an employer to provide information, training and supervision for staff on health and safety matters. Unless he has less than five staff, the employer must provide a statement of general policy on health and safety and arrangements for implementing this. Employees should be consulted about the form and content of this statement.

The HSE discourage the use of 'model' statements. They believe each employer should prepare his own, because anyone who takes the easy option of adopting a 'model' statement is unlikely to give sufficient thought to his policy and its consequences. However, contrary to this advice a specimen format for the written statement is in Box 8.2.

Box 8.2: A specimen written statement on safety

Health and safety in the practice

The partners' policy on health and safety on the surgery premises is to ensure that your working environment is as safe and healthy as possible. As a member of the staff you are expected to support this aim.

Your employer is ultimately responsible for your health and safety; you also have a legal duty to take reasonable care to avoid any action or working pattern which might cause injury to yourself, your colleagues or other people using the surgery premises. In particular, you should not meddle with or misuse any clothing or equipment which has been provided to protect health and safety.

There are certain hazards which you should know about:

1   prams and cycles parked on the premises;
2   medical equipment and instruments used in the consulting rooms;
3   cooking utensils and equipment used in the staff rest room.

You must report any accident to the doctor in charge as soon as possible. You should then write down what has happened, explaining how the accident occurred, so that we can take steps to avoid its repetition.

When a GP prepares his own 'written statement' it should be simple and concise. Long sentences and long words reduce impact. Any safety rules should be clear and comprehensive.

The written statement may be included in each employee's written contract of employment. If it is included it may need to be reviewed and amended from time to time and it must apply to everyone working on the surgery premises. In a small practice, with less than five staff, the statement can be posted in a public place. It is not necessary to give everyone a copy of the written statement.

Safety officers

Safety officers and safety representatives are appointed if an employer recognizes a trade union. In general practice these are most likely to be found in health centres where health authority staff work alongside practice staff.

Staff who are appointed as safety representatives have considerble powers on health and safety matters; inspecting the workplace, enquiring into accidents, raising complaints directly with the GP and insisting on a joint staff – management safety committee being formed. Safety representatives have a legal right to challenge the employer on all matters relating to health and safety.

It has been proposed that safety representatives and safety committees should be appointed where the staff are not unionized. Because both the employer and staff share a legal duty to promote the health and safety of everyone using the premises, the Health and Safety Commission have suggested that both should be involved in developing and promoting health and safety policy and procedures.

A safety committee is simply not possible in a small practice. Instead one member of staff could serve as the 'safety officer' to monitor health and safety. The practice manager may be well suited to do this. However the GPs, as employers, cannot and must not simply pass over their responsibility as employers to the practice manager. They must be involved and the 'safety officer' should report to one of the partners.

Duties to other persons using the premises

While the Health and Safety Act is mostly concerned with the safety of employees an employer also has a duty to ensure the safety of anyone who enters the surgery or health centre. This includes patients, pharmaceutical representatives, visitors, builders, tradesmen and health authority staff.

If the premises are owned by a private landlord or Local Health Authority, the licence or lease may impose this duty upon these other parties who may also be liable if there is an accident.

The Act requires the practice to be organized so as to ensure that all users of the premises are safe from risks of personal injury; for example, it is necessary to consider whether they present any potential hazards to elderly or infirm patients. The Occupier's Liability Act 1957 already lays down a 'common duty of care' owed to all persons using the premises.

Notifying accidents and dangerous occurrences

The Act requires the employer to maintain a record of accidents and, if he is the 'controller of the premises', to notify the HSE of certain serious accidents to anyone on the premises, including staff, patients, workmen or health authority staff.

Normally the employer and controller of the premises will be responsible for any accident. Although there may be circumstances where the owner of the premises and not the GPs will be responsible, it is best to assume that the practice should notify the HSE.

COSHH Regulations

The new Control of Substances Hazardous to Health Regulations 1988 (COSHH) apply new and additional obligations on employers to control hazardous substances and to protect people exposed to them. These Regulations cover virtually all substances hazardous to health. Only those substances covered by their own legislation are excluded, such as asbestos, lead and material producing ionizing radiations. The Regulations set out essential measures that employers (and sometimes employees) have to take. Failure to comply with COSHH, in addition to exposing employees to risk, constitutes an offence and is subject to penalties under the Health and Safety at Work Act 1974. Substances hazardous to health include those labelled as dangerous (i.e. every toxic, harmful, irritant or corrosive) under other statutory requirements.

What are employers required to do?

The basic principles of occupational hygiene underlie the COSHH Regulations. These include:

- assessing the risk to health arising from work and what precautions are needed;
- introducing measures to prevent or control the risk;
- ensuring that control measures are used, equipment is properly maintained and procedures observed;
- monitoring, where necessary, the exposure of employees and carrying out an appropriate form of surveillance of health;
- informing, instructing and training employees about the risks and the precautions to be taken.

All employers need to consider how COSHH applies to their employees and working environment. For most GPs compliance should be simple and straightforward. Several publications giving more detailed information on COSHH and its requirements are available from your local office of the HSE.

The employees' responsibilities

Staff are required to take reasonable care for their own health and safety on the premises, and for the safety of other users of the premises who may be affected by their actions to co-operate with the employer in carrying out these duties.

Although the duties of employees apply 'while at work' it would be wise to assume that these apply throughout the time they remain on the premises. This is important since accidents can occur when staff are preparing tea or lunch in a staff rest room.

Staff must not interfere with or misuse any equipment provided for the purposes of health and safety, such as fire exits, fire extinguishers, and any warning notices. This includes any safety procedures applying to a kitchen cloakroom or rest room.

How is the law enforced?

It is important to remember that the Health and Safety at Work Act is a criminal statute and the HSE an enforcement body. Failure to carry out any duty under the Act constitutes an offence and can lead to a prosecution, fine or imprisonment.

However, the HSE is firmly committed to persuasion. It has discretion to decide whether to prosecute and only does so after careful consideration of advice from the inspector. If a prosecution should arise, the courts would assess what is reasonably practicable in the light of available resources.

Each area of the country has its own inspectors, and one or more of these will be specifically concerned with health service premises, including GP surgeries. Each inspector has considerable powers and these are stated in his warrant of appointment. He may enter any premises to enforce this law, and does not need to seek permission before doing so. However, he can only enter at a 'reasonable time'.

In practice, notice is given of a visit and an inspector will telephone to arrange an appointment. Very rarely 'surprise' inspections are made in response to a complaint from an employee or a user of the premises. Otherwise, the only reason why unannounced visits are made is that the inspector finds that he has some spare time available and includes a visit to a small premises within his organized schedule of visits to larger establishments. Although these 'surprise' visits have caused anxiety, no offence is intended and the inspector should not be suspected of harbouring an ulterior motive.

An inspection

If there are five or more staff, the inspector will wish to see a statement of safety policy and instructions on safety procedures. He will also want to see the accident book.

The inspector will examine the electrical equipment. This should be in good working order and there should be adequate maintenance arrangements. The toilet and washing facilities should be at least equal to those required in offices. In particular, he will probably expect to find a supply of hot and cold running water, and he may even propose elbow-operated taps in all rooms used for examining and treating patients.

There are other matters, including the heating system, drug storage arrangements, steam sterilizers, clinical waste disposal, and heating and lighting standards, which an inspector will also be concerned about.

When he has completed his inspection, the inspector will normally raise directly any improvements required with the person in administrative charge of the surgery. If these matters are not of major importance he will just request that they are carried out as soon as possible.

More serious matters could lead to a formal letter from him, or even a written notice requiring them to be put right within a specified period of time—not less than 21 days. In these circumstances the inspector would also warn the staff of his intention to serve a written notice.

In the most unlikely circumstances of there being a serious risk to health and safety, which should never occur in a GP's surgery, the inspector can issue a prohibition notice. Where there is a very serious risk, all work has to stop immediately.

The accident book

The employer is obliged to keep an accident book, in which all notifiable accidents and occurrences are recorded. This enables the employer to monitor these and take preventive action to avoid any recurrence. A record book is published by the Health and Safety Executive (*Record of Accidents, Dangerous Occurrences and Ill-Health Enquiries*, F2509, HMSO). It is interesting to note that any self-employed person is exempt from this reporting procedure; the GP need not report any accident to himself.

An action list

1   A written statement of policy on health and safety should be issued to all staff, if there are five or more employees. This written statement can be included in the contracts of employment.
2   Keep an accident book and copies of form 2508, the accident report form.
3   Electrical equipment should be regularly maintained and serviced.

4   One member of the staff may be appointed as the 'safety officer'. The practice manager may be best able to take on this responsibility.

5   Any known hazards should be checked at regular intervals to see if improvements need to be made. Obvious examples include loose floor coverings, any building work, electrical plugs and equipment.

6   Patients and visitors should be warned by written notices of any hazards on the premises. This is particularly important if there are building works in progress.

7   The premises' lease of licence agreement should be reviewed. This should state who is responsible for maintaining and repairing the premises. If in doubt, contact the BMA Regional Office.

9 Quality and its Measurement

What is quality?

Like beauty, quality is in the eye of the beholder. It cannot be defined objectively. To a large extent, it depends on the angle from which it is viewed and even then opinions vary. Individual opinion also changes with time. General practice is viewed from several angles including those of the patient, the practice staff, the GPs themselves, hospital-based medical staff and the FHSAs representing the government and the bureaucracy of the health service. All of these groups have a legitimate interest in quality but because they are viewing from different positions, they are interested in different attributes. Some aspects of quality may concern all parties but mostly they relate solely to one and not all of these groups.

The patient's viewpoint

The emphasis here is on personal satisfaction with the service available. He or she wants ready access to the doctor of his choice and anything that interferes with that is seen as detrimental. Delays are especially irksome; those involved in getting an appointment, including telephone difficulties; those involved in barriers at the reception desk (imagined or real); those relating to administrative chores which the patient considers trivial, but for the practice recording system may be essential and even time-consuming. He seeks a reasonable duration of consultation uncluttered by interruptions from the telephone; a feeling of empathy from the doctor; an adequate explanation of his problem and appropriate advice. Patients may also seek their own way—to obtain referral to a specialist when they want it or to be given sleeping tablets or antibiotics when they think they are necessary.

Most of the items which go to make up personal satisfaction are appropriate to assessing quality from whichever position it is viewed, but judgements about therapy and intervention are based on expert knowledge which most patients do not have. You tend to judge shops by the reception and services at the counter and patients will judge practices in the same way.

The practice staff viewpoint

In the organization of the practice, quality starts with adequate availability of doctors. It is not sufficient simply to connect a house to the electricity system, there needs to be an adequate distribution of outlets in the form of power sockets and lights. This principle extends to many aspects of organizing a practice; an adequate number of telephone lines, sufficient seats in the waiting room, sufficient slots in the appointment system, etc. The organization of the practice is seen in its day-to-day working arrangements, the way emergencies are coped with and the availability of the doctor to the reception staff.

The general practitioner's viewpoint

A simple expression of quality for the individual doctor is the avoidance of mistakes, but this expression begs too many questions. There are many types of mistake, some of which can only be identified a long time afterwards. A patient may die at home during convalescence from a heart attack managed at home: the doctor as a consequence (and the relatives) may feel it was a mistake not to have arranged the patient's admission to hospital. Such a 'mistake' may not be due to an incorrect decision at the relevant time since by the same token, a patient recovering in hospital from an uncomplicated heart attack might be considered the result of an inappropriate admission. Every doctor has the conflicting experiences on the one hand of being thanked by relatives in circumstances where he feels he might have done more, and on the other of being criticized where he left no stone unturned.

Although it is a strictly personal opinion, quality is personal satisfaction with the service that I provide. That satisfaction is derived from a conviction that my actions have not entailed unnecessary risk, that they are based on sound evidence and they are not wasteful of resources. These are Utopian ideals and in their entirety, almost impossible to measure. The evaluation of risk is particularly difficult and only rarely is there sufficient evidence to define it in absolute terms. It is accepted that oral contraception with the combined pill is not ideal after the age of 35 years but all the evidence on which that conclusion is based stems from epidemiological studies of contraceptives with higher oestrogen dosage than are used today.

Respect from colleagues (partners, neighbouring doctors, local consultants) is important to most GPs and contributes significantly to the way in which a doctor views the quality of performance. To that end, a GP will seek when referring a patient, not to miss an obvious diagnosis or omit a desirable investigation within his control. Nor will he seek to refer a patient for whom no additional medical opinion or service is required. GPs are very conscious that their performance is open to the judgement of specialist colleagues whenever a referral is made. In a sense however, the converse also applies. The management of a patient in hospital, the delays, seemingly unnecessary tests and the understanding a patient receives of his problem are all used by GPs in assessing the performance of specialists.

It is very hard to deliver a service of good quality if a person is not happy in his role, and that applies to every member of the practice team. Some GPs are very happy in the role of a social psychologist whereas others only feel content in a strictly clinical role. Both positions are acceptable but doctors from these opposing ends of the spectrum have different perceptions of quality. Neither is wrong but in issues of quality, it is difficult to make any comparison between the two.

In order to judge quality in comparative terms, it would be necessary to define the context. The only acceptable definition is the 'contract' or contents of the 'Red Book' in which the GP's role is specified. Mistakes may be judged by failure to comply with these obligations but these minimum standards do nothing to enhance quality in any sense of the word which includes a recognition that standards should be targets to which you aspire and which change with advancing knowledge.

The hospital staff viewpoint

Much attention has been given to the judgements of patients and of colleagues but every doctor in hospital even at very junior level is conscious of the way individual practices are 'judged'. Hospital colleagues are not looking for over-sophisticated diagnoses. Rather, they are concerned with a healthy administrative arrangement in the practice. Can the GPs be contacted easily? Do the records contain a reliable record of prescribed medication? Are recommendations for follow-up care followed? As far as the GP is concerned personally, he will be judged by the quality of his letters and the appropriateness of his referrals and use of the pathology laboratory.

Although practices and hospitals might jointly be concerned in the welfare of individual patients, each can easily become separated and lose sight of the other's veiwpoint. Much can be done to foster good relations by arranging joint clinical meetings. It is here that methods of audit such as random case analysis might operate at their best.

The administrative viewpoint

The FHSA is the administrative arm of the National Health Service controlling general practice. Quality at this level is accurate registration, efficient office procedures, correct form filling, etc.—all aspects of management which to doctors can be the antithesis of care. You should not criticize however; efficient clerical systems are necessary. If a complaint is made against a doctor, it is largely determined according to the minimum standard laid down in the 'Red Book', and accurate clerical details may be an essential part of the doctor's defence.

The recent government White Paper *Working for Patients* proposed certain basic standards of quality in respect of immunization and cervical cytology achievement. Target levels attract bonus payments. There is a new emphasis on preventive care and it is here that the definition of quality is easiest to appreciate. More is better, provided more people are covered by a preventive procedure. More is not better if it means simply that the same people are given more frequent attention.

How can quality be measured?

In this section, a number of methods are considered whereby quality can be assessed within the practice. In general these are concerned with quality of clinical performance although there are many parallels in other aspects of practice activity. The methods described here can be tailored to any practice function.

Random case analysis

Random case analysis involves an evaluation of the management of a particular patient selected at random. It is unnecessary to be over-sophisticated in making the choice. For example an analysis can be made where each of the partners identifies three patients on the appointment list of patients seen by another doctor during the previous week. These are put in a box and extracted at random in a practice meeting. The consultations in question are then discussed. The doctor involved is challenged as to his management, therapeutic action and quality of records.

Random case analysis picks up the best of the clinical case conference familiar to medical students and hospital-based doctors, but avoids that element of showmanship in which the cases discussed were selected to demonstrate impeccable management or aspects of intellectual wizardry prompting the derivation of abstruse diagnoses. Cases selected by random methods are equally likely to reveal weaknesses as strengths. The important points are that every doctor has an equal chance of sitting in the firing line and that the forum for discussion is a group of equals each of whom may be in the hot seat with the next case.

Record review

Record review involves sampling the records for some specific piece of information:

- when did this patient last receive a cytology test?
- when was this patient last seen?
- has this child received his pre-school booster immunization?
- how recent is the last recording of this man's blood pressure?

The entry point for a record review relates to the question on hand. For most purposes, it is perfectly acceptable to take serial entries from the practice recording system, e.g. every fifth record in the filing boxes; every tenth record for each letter of the alphabet up to a maximum of 10 records per letter; serial entries from the appointment list; or from the age–sex register. If necessary, the extraction can be confined to one sex or to a particular age group. It is however important that you achieve a sufficient sample to deal with the task in hand and this aspect will be discussed later.

Activity analyses

The simplest form of activity analyses involve the use of score grids (as illustrated in Fig. 9.1). A score is made as an event occurs. In most such analyses, the exercise is conducted over a specific period, e.g. two or four weeks. For some activities, it is more appropriate to continue the scoring exercise until a specified minimum number of events has occurred. The activity in question may relate to the performance of the practice, individual doctor or individual staff member.

The method can be criticized because the act of measuring performance may induce us to behave differently. Such criticism cannot be denied but it should be viewed against the great economy of effort which this method entails.

The prescribing audit of the Prescription Pricing Authority is an example of an activity analysis which is government-sponsored. This is primarily a measure of practice performance because it does not present prescribing rates for the individual partners in a way which permits detailed comparison between them. In it, the various measurements of prescribing within the practice are presented against a background of local information about other practices. You have to recognize however that this report tells you nothing about quality. Using these data, individual doctors may make inferences about quality but their perceptions of quality are individual and to a large extent reflect their own prejudices. One doctor looking at a low prescribing rate for psycho-active drugs may pat himself on the back because it is fashionable to criticize these drugs. Another with a high

A score is made on each occasion an antibiotic or sulphonamide drug is prescribed for systemic use, as a new course of treatment in an episode of illness. Prescriptions which simply continue a course of treatment without a change of antibiotic prescribed are not scored. A score should be made however where a course of treatment is initiated in circumstances in which no fact to face consultation occurred.

	0 – 4 years	5 – 14 years	15 – 64 years	65 + years
Natural penicillins eg. Pen. V. Pen. G.	1 2 3 4 5 6 7 8 9 10 11 12 13 14 15 16 17 18 19 20	1 2 3 4 5 6 7 8 9 10 11 12 13 14 15 16 17 18 19 20	1 2 3 4 5 6 7 8 9 10 11 12 13 14 15 16 17 18 19 20	1 2 3 4 5 6 7 8 9 10 11 12 13 14 15 16 17 18 19 20
Broad spectrum & other penicillins eg. ampicillin.	1 2 3 4 5 6 7 8 9 10 11 12 13 14 15 16 17 18 19 20	1 2 3 4 5 6 7 8 9 10 11 12 13 14 15 16 17 18 19 20	1 2 3 4 5 6 7 8 9 10 11 12 13 14 15 16 17 18 19 20	1 2 3 4 5 6 7 8 9 10 11 12 13 14 15 16 17 18 19 20
Erythromycins	1 2 3 4 5 6 7 8 9 10	1 2 3 4 5 6 7 8 9 10	1 2 3 4 5 6 7 8 9 10	1 2 3 4 5 6 7 8 9 10
Tetracyclines	1 2 3 4 5 6 7 8 9 10 11 12 13 14 15	1 2 3 4 5 6 7 8 9 10 11 12 13 14 15	1 2 3 4 5 6 7 8 9 10 11 12 13 14 15	1 2 3 4 5 6 7 8 9 10 11 12 13 14 15
Sulphonamides	1 2 3 4 5	1 2 3 4 5	1 2 3 4 5	1 2 3 4 5
Co-trimoxazole drugs eg. Septrin	1 2 3 4 5 6 7 8 9 10	1 2 3 4 5 6 7 8 9 10	1 2 3 4 5 6 7 8 9 10	1 2 3 4 5 6 7 8 9 10
Others	1 2 3 4 5	1 2 3 4 5	1 2 3 4 5	1 2 3 4 5

Summarize the above results in the grid below:

Age	0 – 4 yrs	5 – 14 yrs	15 – 64 yrs	64 + yrs
Natural penicillins				
Broad spectrum & other penicillins				
Erythromycins				
Tetracyclines				
Sulphonamides				
Co-trimoxazole				
Others				

Figure 9.1　A practice activity score grid: choice of chemotherapy.

prescribing rate may feel satisfied that he is sensitive to the psychiatric aspects of illness and reasonably consider that his patients are, on balance, helped by these drugs.

However many limitations and however much it can be criticized, the arrival of prescribing information in this form should be regarded as a milestone in the field of quality control. It provides that most essential ingredient—objective and reproducible information about *what is going on.* Information which is irrefutable and not simply an opinion about what is going on.

Standardized protocols

The emergence of acceptable and standardized protocols is also an advance. Although many of them are not perfect, they provide a framework of reference for consistent measurement. Generally speaking, you should accept tested and standardized protocols but measurements of compliance with them can involve differential analysis of specific points with which a practice may disagree.

Standardized protocols can of course be practice-based and a primary object of practice activity analysis is the development of procedural protocols. Such protocols can be designed not only for examining clinical management, but also for basic practice procedures. For example, a procedural protocol could be established to define how the appointment list is to be scheduled to accommodate the absence of a partner on holiday.

Patient questionnaires

Patient questionnaires have a particular place in assessing satisfaction. Care should be taken however not to confuse patient satisfaction with good clinical care. For clinical reasons, it may be desirable for a patient to attend for clinical review rather than receive a repeat prescription but this requirement may upset him and make him dissatisfied.

The nature of standards

The nub of quality control lies in the nature and definition of standards. The fact that there are so few unequivocal standards makes this difficult. Standards can be defined for administrative procedures: they can also be defined for preventive care where a greater coverage is always better. In clinical practice however, they arise from subjective opinions: opinions about the diagnosis, the severity of symptoms and the management. The differentiation between earache and otitis media is extremely difficult.

Many studies purport to study otitis media but there is little scientific work on 'earache'. Standards of care can only be specified for patients with otitis media if you first agree which patients with earache are not suffering from otitis media.

Perhaps the most important point to make here is that standards must be derived from real data. Standards derived from discussions tend to be unrealistic. Aspirations are so much higher than achievements that without the corrective of observed performance, you are apt to think yourselves better than you really are. Unrealistic targets lead to 'failure in the examination' and you tend to stop taking the examination if you keep failing.

Two possibilities exist when standards are based on measured data. The measurement itself can define the standard. In the Prescription Pricing Authority analysis of prescribing, the average cost for the local area defines a standard or 'norm'. Alternatively the measurement of existing perform-ance allows us to define a target. From his prescribing report, a GP may decide that he is using more drugs of one particular type than he feels is desirable. That decision is based on the real information available in the report but is not necessarily anything to do with the practice comparison with local average. The decision here concerns the direction of quality. In the judgement of quality, the standard is sometimes only discernible in the direction in which we seek to move.

Perhaps even more important than the exercise of standard setting is the willingness to examine ourselves. Ideally this should be done with real information and in the presence of colleagues who have also measured their own performance. It is in this dialogue that you derive standards that are attainable and realistic and it is here also that you learn about ways of coping with problems which have been successfully dealt with by others. The fact that one of your colleagues has achieved a goal, target or standard to which you ascribe, is the stimulus you need in the pursuit of quality.

Samples and sample size

Although this book does not address the mathematical issues surrounding sampling theory, it is impossible to understand measurements of perform-ance without having some appreciation of the techniques of sampling and the adequacy of samples. If a judgement is required about some element of performance, let us say home visiting, then you have to be confident that you have studied an adequate sample of home visits from which you can draw conclusions. Suppose Dr A thought that he visited patients more frequently than Dr B and wished to demonstrate that fact. If indeed Dr A made an average of 30 visits a week and Dr B 10, the difference would be quite clear over only two or three weeks of study. If however the difference was more like 22 and 18 visits a week respectively, it would be necessary to go on for several weeks before feeling satisfied that a true difference existed. Our sample therefore relates to the degree of difference you seek to identify. The larger the sample the greater the confidence you can have in the result.

As a rule of thumb, if you propose to measure some aspect of performance or to obtain information about a group of patients with a particular problem, a minimum of 30 must be studied before you can have any degree of confidence in the results of your analyses. Such a sample will identify a difference of 50% between two recorders but will not reliably identify a difference of 20%. If in a practice audit information is required about male and female persons separately, then 30 patients of each sex must be studied.

Ideally, samples should be taken at random or a sampling method employed such that a representative sample is recruited. Representation in this context may involve ensuring that samples are drawn in a way which includes every doctor in the practice and every day of the week. For most practice purposes you do not need to be submerged by the complexities of recruiting a completely random sample but you should always take care to take samples which are not obviously biased. For some purposes, consecutive cases are an acceptable sample. A legitimate assumption can be made that within 30 cases recruited consecutively, there will be an appropriate mixture of events occurring by chance that the total of 30 is satisfactory. This of course could not be the case if you deliberately chose to study home visits during an influenza epidemic, or at other atypical times.

Comparability

If you are to derive practice statistics that can be used for comparison, either between people or between practices or between similar events separated in time, then you have to present your information as rates. A rate requires a numerator and a denominator. Ideally numerators and denominators should be 'equivalent'. The most useful denominator in general practice is the practice registered population. Since the denominator is of persons, then so should be the numerator. This can be a counsel of perfection because counting methods which record events are much simpler than methods which record persons. You can count home visits much more easily than counting persons who are visited at home. This distinction though theoretically valid, is unnecessarily detailed for most audits in general practice. The interpretation of data based on events in practice as opposed to persons will rarely differ from the viewpoint of the practical observer such as the general practitioner or the practice manager. However, you must not lose sight of the difference since if you wish to apply statistical tests to evaluate difference such details are critical. The use of statistical methods based on rank order offers a solution to this problem.

There are several potential denominators for practice audit. The first is the group under study. We could, for example, look at the distribution of home visits undertaken by a doctor simply by expressing them in percentages in age and sex groups. This would tell him nothing about his overall visiting rate but it would be very clear if he were visiting a disproportionate number of elderly persons. Secondly, you can use total consultations. Home visits expressed as a percentage of consultations within age and sex groups is a useful practice statistic and in addition it can be applied to an individual doctor. A totalled number of consultations is used extensively in practice activity analysis because it is the easiest denominator for use with data based on individual GPs. The total number of persons consulting is theoretically a better denominator because a person is a unit with more meaning than a consultation (one person may make 0, 1, 2 or several consultations). Though this is probably the best denominator for measuring practice activity it is not easy to obtain because linkage must be retained in the recording system such that individual patients are consistently identified. To date, this has not been realistic but the advent of practice computers will change all that. Finally, the practice registered list: this is the denominator used for presenting prescribing data but it only has a useful meaning for the practice and not for individual doctors, excepting only where doctors manage a personalized list, yet operate within a partnership, (an arrangement which is very rarely achieved). The practice list is subject to list inflation which is a small but relevant criticism of this denominator.

When analysing or presenting practice data, it is desirable that the recognized age groups for epidemiological study are employed. These are 0–4, 5–14, 15–24, 25–44, 45–64, 65–74, 75+ years. For many purposes, practices may chose to present data with some of these groups combined, e.g. 25–64 and 65+ years—a procedure which is permissible. It is however unwise to generate your own group divisions as there will be reduced opportunities for comparison with other work. The age groups under 1 year and 5–15 are sometimes used in addition to those mentioned above.

Standardization

Standardization procedures can be made to assist comparability. For example, let us go back to the study of home visits in which Dr A made 22 visits a week and Dr B 18. Let us suppose that these two doctors had studied their visiting pattern for 10 weeks and concluded that Dr A did indeed make more visits than Dr B. By way of explanation, Dr B might allege that although there was a difference in the actual number of visits undertaken, the underlying behaviour of the two doctors was the same; Dr A simply made more visits because he looked after more elderly people. The derivation of a standardized visiting ratio would be a means whereby the visiting patterns of both doctors could be compared as though the two doctors looked after populations of similar age and sex composition. In careful analyses of differences, it is necessary to bear age and sex standardization in mind but for practical purposes, in most GP audits, it is unnecessary. It certainly would not have been necessary in the example where Dr A made 30 visits and Dr B 10.

The presentation and assessment of practice data

Doctors are usually very good at collecting data. The problem commonly seen is that they collect it in a manner that is unique and it is very hard retrospectively to make comparisons. If in a practice you wish to examine some aspect of performance, it is worth searching the library for a method that someone else has tested and is already using. Although the very simple practice activity analysis score grids cannot provide very detailed analysis of individual practice problems, they have been used by many doctors and there is now a useful and available data bank for comparison.

Data for use in practice and group meetings must show in a simple manner the actual performance of an individual doctor and relate it to the group average. Ideally, the individual performance should be confidential to that one observer. Where possible, data should be presented in a good visual manner—a histogram is often more useful than a table. All necessary data should be available to facilitate interpretation. In the series of analysis published as Practice Activity Analysis, the results usually included the rate of consultations per 1000 list during the study period. (The derivation of the list for this purpose is very approximate and involved averaging the total list between the partners.) An extreme value for this particular statistic is a warning to an individual doctor to think very carefully about his consultation pattern during the period of survey before interpreting the results for the main analysis.

When sharing the results, the best discussions come from groups 8 to 12 strong, containing doctors from more than one practice and a group in which all the members have participated in the data collection exercise. Contributions from doctors who have not measured their own performance are not welcome on these occasions. The groups need to be led by someone who is familiar with data of this type and who is convinced of the merits of self-evaluation in groups. It is easy to be destructive because data collected in this way is inevitably weak when it comes to statistical manipulation. However, when considering personal performance, only very occasionally will an individual have an apparently misleading notion of his own performance. If you were to pursue practice analyses to the point at which you could be confident that no one would ever be misled, you would have to use much larger samples and reconsider the question of the appropriate denominator. This may well come, as computer technology advances, but for the time being, we must be content with the systems that are available and not defer the issue of quality control until it is foisted upon us by governments.

When considering some area of performance, it helps considerably if someone first considers the data as a whole and formulates topical questions which can be addressed in the discussion.

Practice reports

Practices are now required to produce an annual prctice report. Certain aspects of practice activity are prescribed, but there are benefits in extending the range of activities for analysis. The report should not be seen simply as a historical record because it can also provide a pointer to future strategy. In fact, a key element is the opportunity it provides to identify matters requiring attention and desirable targets to achieve in the following year.

The production of practice reports is not a new function; many practices have regarded it as an aspect of good management for many years. Practice managers are usually willing to share their methods of analysis with others less experienced, and further advice can be obtained from the FHSA or Health Board. The principle can be readily understood by studying the annual reports that limited companies produce for their shareholders.

Information to be provided in practice report

Staff

- Total number of staff (but not their names).
- Principle duties of each employee and hours worked each week.
- Qualifications of each employee.
- Relevant training undertaken by employee in last 5 years.

Practice premises

- Any variations in floor space, design or quality since the last annual report.
- Any variations anticipated in the next 12 months.

Referral of patients

- Total number referred as in-patients.
- Total number referred as out-patients.

- Total referred for each specialty and hospital concerned: general surgical, general medical, orthopaedic, rheumatology (physical medicine), ear, nose and throat, gynaecology, obstetrics, paediatrics, ophthalmology, psychiatry, geriatrics, dermatology, neurology, genitourinary, X-ray, pathology and others (including plastic surgery, accident and emergency and endocrinology).
- Total number of patients referred by themselves (if known) and to which service.

Doctor's commitments

- A description of any posts held, including hourly commitment.
- A description of all work undertaken, including hourly commitment.

Patient participation

- Any arrangements whereby the practice receives patients comments on the services provided.

Drugs and appliances

- Does the practice have its own formulary?
- Does the doctor use a separate formulary?
- The doctor's arrangements for repeat prescriptions.

10 Audit and the Practice Manager

THE previous chapter has spelt out some of the principles behind quality control and some methods by which it can be achieved. In this chapter you will consider some more specific examples of audit and how practices will be involved. The Government's document *Working for Patients*, published in 1989, placed great emphasis on audit in the health service and this was one of the few elements of the White Paper that met with almost unanimous professional support.

There is a requirement for all doctors to demonstrate that they are taking part in medical audit and GPs will be encouraged in this by the establishment in each FHSA area (and by other bodies in Scotland and Northern Ireland) of a Medical Audit Advisory Group (MAAG).

There have been a number of attempts to define what is meant by medical audit and one simple definition is 'looking at what we do to see if we can do it better'. This is an activity which is not peculiar to doctors in the practice team and it is one which you all should be, and usually have been, engaged in.

Attitudes

You should recognize at the start that medical audit is a potentially threatening activity for all who take part in it. There is an implication which you could all admit privately that what you are doing is not always the best that could be done. Whilst it is reasonable to admit this to yourselves privately it is not so easy to admit it to others or, more alarming still, to have it pointed out by others. Yet we are all working for the same objectives and desire to provide the best possible care for our patients. If you can somehow get rid of the attitude that it is blameworthy to identify a deficiency then you are half way to developing the sort of personal confidence and mutual respect of others that is an indispensable condition for medical audit. This change of attitude is the first important step to take. It is easier to do it within a group of equals – peer group – who work together, so the doctors in a practice may find it easier to start amongst themselves than have other staff members involved. Similarly, a group of practice nurses may find it easier to set out on the exercise without doctors being present. As confidence in the method develops it is possible to extend audit to others working in different practices or coming from different fields of work. It will be seen that confidentiality is an important feature of this exercise for if you are unable to be truthful then you are unable to conduct honest audit.

There is, of course, one other attitude that is important. All those who take part must see the exercise as being important and relevant to them in their work or, at any rate, in the work of the practice as a whole. They should understand that audit is a very powerful educational tool and if carried out properly one of the most important agencies for change that exists. For this reason the choice of audit topic is important and should be the choice of all.

Resources

The most precious resource you have is time. This has become even more obvious recently when a wide range of new activities have been thrust upon general practice. When you are busy it may seem too much to ask for an extra hour or two each week for medical audit and yet if you do not do it the quality of work may deteriorate, dangerous mistakes may occur and you may become even more busy for audit may reveal ways of saving time or using time more effectively. It is therefore a priority activity.

The second resource you need is access to good data. Here another important principle operates, the data used for audit should be based on that required for the normal clinical care of patients or the management of the practice. Examples of this would include the clinical notes of patients, letters sent and received, emergency calls, appointments, PACT data and so on. It is a good general rule that if, in order to carry out an audit you have to set up and collect entirely new data that you do not normally need or use, think again.

Types of audit

Critical event audit

There are two broad groups of audit subjects. The first, and the one which is most familiar is critical event audit. You will be familiar with the discussion that takes place, often in an informal setting over coffee, in which the problems faced by a single doctor in the care of a patient are raised. The issues raised, may be of a patient who fails to respond to treatment or advice, or angry relatives of a patient who died, and the doctor or nurse gets support, alternative suggestions or new perspectives from the group. Critical event audit disciplines this informal activity and takes it further for it asks not only what might be better done in relation to this case but what lessons might be learnt from this case that are of general application. It tries to develop a standard of care from the particular against which the care of the many can be measured.

For example, a young woman in the practice who is under treatment for depression commits suicide. You might enquire what clues, if any, existed for this behaviour and how could they have been identified. You might ask what preventive measures exist, what other services are used and what are their deficiencies. You might, in fact learn from this single case a pattern of activity which is better than you had before. From this you can begin to create a standard of care which you can test on other cases. It might contain a number of criteria, or factors which produce a more accurate definition of what is meant by 'depressed', what you should record, what you should do for continuity of care, how you should communicate, what and how should be prescribed and so on. This type of audit has the attraction that you do not need large numbers of cases before you can do it better! It also emphasizes the fact that such standards are not unchangeable. They are not written on tablets of stone. As another such audit is done your standards may change for new drugs or new patterns of care may come along. Audit is essentially a dynamic process and should never be static.

Whilst you should not decry the value of this sort of audit, and carried out in a rigorous way it can produce effective change, most of the time when you think of medical audit you think of the sort of data described in the previous chapter. The fact that all participants in audit must feel committed to the importance and relevance of the topic has already been mentioned. This is particularly important in this form of audit when the data collected is the result of others work. An example of this might be a decision to audit some aspects of the care of asthma.

Discussion of this within the practice might lead the doctors to decide that they need a register of all the asthmatics in the practice. They know from other studies how many asthmatics might be expected in their population and the practice should be able to identify a number approximately to this. From this the question might arise that if there is a difference why is this so? Are all the asthmatics being identified?

The practice might decide that a peak flow measurement, or several measurements should be included in each asthmatic's notes; that the current medication should be easily identifiable, that those on regular therapy should be seen at least every three months, that prophylactic treatment should have been considered for each patient and so on. These criteria lead to the definition of a *standard* of care and with the list of asthmatics it should be possible to extract from the notes information about each of these criteria. You might then report to the practice meeting:

Number of asthmatics with peak flow recorded within the past three years	= 47%
Number with medication clearly recorded	= 88%
Number seen in past three months	= 17%

Consideration of this simple data allows the practice to reconsider whether the criterion is appropriate and if not what should replace it. It also allows the practice to take steps to meet the criteria which are thought to be correct.

You cannot audit everything. If the practice decides to look at the care of asthma does that mean that the care of diabetes and hypertension is neglected? Not necessarily so, but there is a danger of producing a programme of care that is unbalanced and it needs people with the ability to take a broad view to decide that 'paying Peter might mean robbing Paul', that the investment of too much time and energy in asthma clinics might not leave enough for other equally important topics.

In this type of audit the practice manager has an important role. Firstly, it is more appropriate for doctors to spend their time establishing the standard of clinical care than physically waste their time collecting all the data. Furthermore, if changes are made as a result of setting standards, for example, that all patients on regular medication for asthma should be reviewed at four-monthly intervals, it would then be the practice manager's task to devise a system for monitoring the effect of changes made.

This introduces another concept, that of the audit cycle (*see* Fig. 10.1). It is necessary to establish recall systems, or check lists in a system that works to those standards, but unless performance is then measured against these standards, the audit cycle fails. Are you, having done this work, actually seeing all your asthmatics on regular medication every four months and if not why not? It might be that you need new criteria and every six months would be more appropriate.

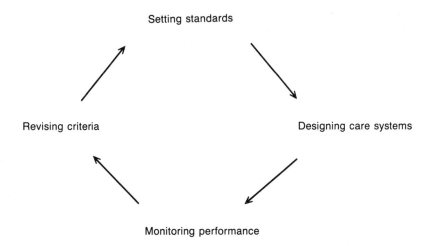

Figure 10.1 The audit cycle.

Auditing the organization

Although supporting medical audit will be an important task for you and your staff it is audit of the organization which will be your most central role. As the expectations of the public increase and we move into an increasingly consumerist society patients identify the standards of general practice with those they might expect from any other service organization. The concepts that you apply to 'service', availability, accessibility, courtesy and good manners, speed and reliability are all applied to general practice. The days when status, mystique and self-importance could be used to conceal failings in these areas have, quite rightly, long gone. There is now an additional concept to bring to the service you provide, that of effectiveness, one subset of which is cost-effectiveness. Much that is done in medicine has a slender base of scientific proof which makes it more important that when you feel on relatively secure ground you should be efficient and effective. This leads you into a more pro-active pattern of behaviour where you seek to prevent disease in a population you are responsible for or to identify disease at an early stage when treatment might be more effective. It also means that continuity of care has to be applied with greater rigour. You are no longer satisfied to record the non-attendance of a patient or even, not be aware of it. You assume that it might be due to your poor communication and seek to ensure that it is at least an informed refusal to attend.

The subset of cost-effectiveness has become more important as the finite nature of your resources becomes more apparent. Just as you can 'rob Peter to pay Paul' in terms of time, so you can by injudicious expenditure of resources upon one patient or one group of patients. All these activities and concepts are affected by the organization and are the concern of the practice manager. To them you can apply the same categories of audit, critical event audit, qualitative analysis, and audit of collected data, quantitative analysis. The same principles apply to each as to when you consider examples of medical audit.

Critical event audit

A patient telephones a request for a visit at 9.15 a.m. on Monday morning. The visit is eventually done at 4.30 p.m. in response to an angry call from a relative. It may, of course, be that the visit was urgent, the patient had appendicitis and seven hours later was more seriously ill. It may be that a hospital doctor commented that 'it would have been so much better if the patient had been seen earlier'. It might even be that a patient dies. Yet it might equally well be someone known to panic about trivia who is actually complaining of a minor rash. Whatever it is it leaves an annoyed patient and relatives who had a perception of urgency, an irritable, tired doctor and, perhaps bruised and guilty staff. It could be dealt with by blaming it all on the patient, 'she never explained what was wrong', 'she could always ring again', 'that was the day we had two doctors off sick', and so on. It could be dealt with much more constructively by using the episode as a critical event audit to create standards that can later be monitored. Is the message recording system adequate? Are the correct questions asked of patients? Should telephone requests be put through to doctors? How are doctors informed? Do we have a system of informing patients about delays? Is it necessary to monitor our response time? What would be the standards against which you measure your performance in all this? Lastly, and most importantly how can you explore these issues with staff so that they feel supported and encouraged rather than bruised and blamed?

Suitable topics for critical event audit might include:

- a confrontation at the reception desk;
- a complaint;
- a medical emergency in the practice when no doctor is available;
- a wrong prescription/note given out;
- a breach of confidentiality.

Collected data audit

The previous chapter has provided examples of some of the ways in which you can use collected data for medical audit. It is just as possible, and important, to collect data about the organization for audit. One example might be to audit the waiting time of patients in the waiting room. Before appointment systems patients seemed to be prepared to wait without complaint to see the doctor, but once appointments were introduced there is a growing impatience as the time extends beyond the point when the patient has been told they will be seen. Much of this waiting time is unnecessary and is due to inefficient organization though, of course, the unexpected may always intervene. Doctors are curiously predictable in the average length of consultations. Some work at an average of 10 minutes and some at 12 or more. Some are much shorter. To make a similar appointment time for every doctor predetermines that some will always be lagging behind. It is possible to work this out in order to prevent predictable delay. If a receptionist notes the time of arrival of a patient, the time seen and the length of a consultation for several sessions of a doctor's consultation serious data will be collected showing the average waiting time and the average length of a consultation and this will allow a pattern to be identified and a standard set which can later be monitored (*see* Fig. 10.2), e.g. so that no

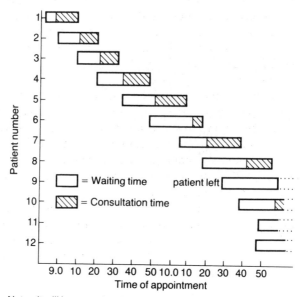

Note: It will be seen that the doctor started four minutes late. His
average consultation time was 12½ minutes and he only
regained part of the lost 30 minutes because one patient left.

Figure 10.2 An audit of waiting time in the surgery (with 10 minute appointments for each patient).

one should want longer than 15 minutes, except when an emergency occurs and the average waiting time should be five minutes. Later audit shows how close to this standard you have come.

Other suitable topics for collected data audit of the organization might include:

- ease/difficulty of telephone access to the surgery;
- time taken to get an appointment;
- repeat prescription system;
- use of investigation services;
- written communication to and from the surgery;
- completeness of claims submitted;
- completeness of payment for claims submitted.

Staff appraisal

This topic is included because, whilst it is not strictly audit, it is part of the same philosophy. Most large organizations are now adopting appraisal systems in which every member of staff is interviewed, usually annually, in a standard and formulated way. The interviews aim to identify the perceived strengths and weaknesses of the staff member, to identify their wishes and objectives for the next year's work and set down a plan that can be reviewed at the end of the year to see how much was achieved. It is therefore a form of 'self-audit' aided by a senior. The practice manager should see each member of staff in privacy and in an undisturbed setting for approximately half an hour. It has been found in practice to be a valuable means by which the practice manager gets to know her staff, a non-threatening way in which staff can talk about any difficulties they might have and any educational needs they perceive.

The plan to deal with these can then be agreed by both and written down to be produced a year later for reappraisal. It needs to be handled sensitively and should be viewed by all as a positive, supportive exercise. It has been shown to be a useful contribution towards maintaining staff morale.

11 Managing Money

Introduction: the practice manager as financial controller

One of the more important tasks of the practice manager is the control of the finances of the practice, ensuring that these are run in an efficient and systematic manner, maximizing the practice income, keeping a control on expenditure and hence increasing the profitability of the practice, not only for the benefit of the doctors but hopefully for the practice manager herself.

In these next sections of studies you will look at several aspects of the manager's role as the financial controller of the practice. If one makes an analogy with the small limited trading company, the role is probably roughly equivalent to that of company secretary or finance director. It is one of huge responsibility; the modern medical practice may well have a turnover running into several hundred thousands of pounds. Practices with a turnover in excess of half a million pounds are now becoming common-place; although the writer has not personally seen a practice with a turnover in excess of one million pounds, its advent cannot be too far away. This responsibility can be expected to increase with the introduction of budgets for the larger practices. We do not consider here the personal aspects of general practice as they affect the doctors and partners themselves. Thus the subject of personal income tax, pensions and retirement, personal financing, etc. are not covered (and should be read in their proper context in the book *Making Sense of Practice Finance* by John Dean, published by Radcliffe Medical Press).

It is also essential that, having read this book and attended the courses, you keep your knowledge up to date.

There are numerous changes in general practice finance, arising not only from the introduction of the GP fund-holding initiative but also from far-reaching changes in the 1990 GP Contract. These are not taken into account in this section, so long as some element of uncertainty continues.

Some of the manager's duties will concern employment; the hiring and firing of staff; payment of wages, etc. This will involve calculation of wages and salaries, a knowledge of PAYE and Class I National Insurance and this is described in that section.

One of the prime arts of management is the successful delegation of responsibility and the manager in general practice must be prepared to, where necessary, ensure that at least some part of her workload is delegated to more junior staff, whom it will be more cost effective to employ for that purpose.

Profitability and how to ensure it

General practice is a business, just like that of the dentist or the chemist or, outside the health care field, the normal conventional trader who buys goods and sells them for profit. They all have one thing in common: the profitable business will normally be the efficient one, and vice versa, although, of course, there is not necessarily a complete correlation between efficiency and the quality of patient care. In general medical practice this can be readily seen by those of us who have the opportunity to compare practices. It is by no means unusual to find two apparently identical practices, with similar numbers of patients and practising from very similar catchment areas, offering the same type of service and with similar numbers of partners, generating entirely different levels of income.

These discrepancies in income levels from general practice are both numerous and legendary. On the one hand, one may find a highly efficient dispensing practice with numbers of outside appointments; probably some private patient work, with maximum staff levels, and the partners earning incomes in excess of £50 000 per annum. This will be a highly efficient business operation, with the partners all taking a share of responsibility for administration and the practice manager dealing with the day-to-day running of the practice, leaving the doctors largely to concentrate on their clinical duties to the ultimate benefit of patients. At the other end of the scale, one comes across an apparently similar practice, with the partners having little interest in administration, probably operating on a shoestring with two or three part-time receptionists, little attention being made to maximize item-of-service claims and with a general air of decay and lack of attention. In this practice the partners may well earn no more than £20 000—far less than even the intended average remuneration in general practice.

Although these are two extreme cases and are merely quoted to illustrate the point, they are by no means untypical of the situation in general practice today. It is often the quality of the practice manager who makes such a difference between two such examples.

If, then, you accept that efficiency equals profitability, how can you assure this efficiency and hence maximize the practice profits? For financial efficiency, a number of criteria are basic and necessary:

1   maximization of income from item-of-service fees;
2   achievement of targets;
3   level of income from promotion clinics;

4   an adequate level of income from non-FHSA sources (*see* p. 147);
5   an economic cost structure, including up-to-date budgeting techniques (*see* 'Control of outgoings');
6   an effective bookkeeping system (*see* 'Basic bookkeeping');
7   a proper control of cash flow, including drawings systems (*see* 'Systems of drawings');
8   an interest and affinity with finance and administration by some or all of the partners.

These eight criteria will not automatically and of themselves create a highly profitable practice where none previously existed, but they will go a great deal of the way towards achieving it and give a foundation upon which to build.

Self-employment and the independent contractor status

The GP is a self-employed businessman, just as is his fellow professional, the solicitor or the architect, or the man running the high street shop. Unfortunately many doctors, starting their careers as they do as employees of a hospital authority, never see themselves as truly self-employed in every sense of the word, looking upon themselves as employees either of their practice or the health authority. This is far from being the case; the jealously-guarded status of the GP (and his colleague in the dental service) as independent contractors dates back to the formation of the NHS in 1948, when the status was negotiated on the GPs' behalf and, apart from one or two occasions over the years when it has seriously been questioned, has stood the test of time.

This section has described what the term 'independent contractor' means. Why is it financially beneficial for the GPs? Let us have a look at this in some detail (*see* Box 11.1).

The advantages

A secured source of income

Unlike his colleagues in other professions, the NHS GP does not have to go out and look for clients (or, in his case, patients); they will come to him and he will normally have little difficulty, unless there is something radically wrong with his practice, in maintaining a standard list size. Indeed, in certain expanding areas, the list may increase at a fairly steady rate and the number of partners in the practice will normally be geared to such factors as the list size in order to ensure an adequate per capita level of income.

The receipt of a regular cheque at the end of each month and each quarter will help to ensure an even cash flow throughout the practice and the GP is saved the time and expense, which is common in other businesses, of having to run complex credit control systems in order to ensure that bills are paid within a reasonable period.

Box 11.1: The NHS GP as independent contractor

Advantages

Schedule D tax status
Occupational pension scheme
Freedom from fee collection
No top limit on earnings
The security of regular income

Obligations

Income enhancement by efficient claims system
Necessity for running an efficient business
Desirability of efficient accounting records
Requirement to employ ancillary staff

Direct and indirect refunds of expenses

The manner in which refunds of expenditure, either by direct payment from the FHSA or by the system of indirect refund of expenses through the Review Body Award, is unique to general practice.

Pensions and superannuation

The NHS superannuation scheme, with proper advice, will give the GP an adequate income and lump sum on retirement. As a result of highly successful negotiations over the years, this has built-in factors such as dynamizing; index-linking; death in service benefits and other matters which are not normally found elsewhere.

Doctors (and their dentist colleagues) are the only people in the country who are both self-employed and members of an occupational pension scheme, in itself an advantage which can carry even further opportunities of enhancing their retirement income.

Taxation

GPs have the facility of being able to pay income tax under Schedule 'D', rather than by the Schedule 'E' status of an employee. The manner in which the respective tax schedules are administered ensures that the GP is considerably better off financially through paying tax as a self-employed professional.

The disadvantages

On the other hand, there are disadvantages as well. One rarely finds in this world that advantages of the nature outlined above are obtained without obligations in return and so it is with GPs.

Outside control of one's income

Just as the GP has a large element of security of his income, so he must accept the fact that, to a large degree, this is determined by an outside body, i.e. the Review Body. Again, this bears little comparison with his outside professional colleagues who are able to sell their own services at whatever fee they consider reasonable and economic, dependent only upon competition and market forces. The typical GP, excepting the relatively modest extra income he may obtain from non-NHS sources, is unable to do this and to a large degree is dependent on the annual remuneration award to determine the level of his income.

Control of staff

He will be responsible for the staffing of his surgery; hiring and firing of employees, calculation of salaries and all that this implies. Many GPs find themselves unable to deal adequately with staffing problems and this should ideally be delegated to the practice manager.

The responsibility of running a business

Most GPs experience continual difficulty, not only in running the business operation of their practice, but in the necessary contact they will have from time to time with other professions, such as accountants, lawyers, bank managers, etc. Without a proper business training they find themselves at a considerable disadvantage and in extreme cases it is not unknown for a young GP to seek to continue his career elsewhere, rather than subjecting himself to pressures of this nature.

In the properly organized general practice, an efficient and capable practice manager will take most, if not all, of these burdens from the shoulders of her doctors.

The Red Book and levels of fee income

The practice manager who wishes to take her duties seriously and to act in the best interest of her doctors, should familiarize herself as best she can with the statement of fees and allowances (SFA) – known universally as 'The Red Book'. Supplied to all GPs in practice, the Red Book is the authoritative work on practice finance. Reference should be sought there for interpretation of any questions on practice finance.

The Red Book is a mine of information and a fully up-to-date amended copy should be available in every surgery. FHSAs issue amendments at fairly regular intervals throughout the year and care should be taken to see that the Red Book is always kept up-to-date for readily obtainable information. It has to be said, however, that it is not perhaps the most readable document. Fortunately, there are a supply of booklets, some of them published by the medical newspapers, which interpret the Red Book and again the conscientious practice manager should ensure that she keeps up-to-date with developments as they arise.

Making Sense of the New Contract, edited by John Chisholm and published by Radcliffe Medical Press, explains fees and allowances in a rather more readable form. Further reading is set out in the 'Financial information' section on page 194.

Fees and allowances payable to GPs are calculated each year and included in the annual Review Body Award. The 21st Review Body Report was published in February 1991 and sets out fees and allowances payable during the year ending 31 March 1992. A list of these fees and allowances is given in Appendix A.

What is far less often appreciated is the basis upon which intended remuneration levels are calculated. Each year the Review Body conducts a statistical sampling process, based upon practice accounts submitted to the Inland Revenue for income tax purposes. The accounts used in this review are restricted; at best they exclude any accounts not ending within the March quarter of each year; accounts prepared on a cash basis and those from practices in Northern Ireland are excluded also. This sampling process, not unlike a 'Gallup Poll' principle, extracts information from a variety of practices selected at random from these accounts available to the Inland Revenue. From this is prepared a calculation of expenses which in turn are converted to an average for a typical practice, and this then includes the element of indirect expenses refund included within GPs' remuneration.

It follows from this process that it is very much to the advantage of GPs as a whole that their accounts show the true level of their expenditure. In many cases, accounts are prepared and submitted which show expenditure 'netted-out' against the direct refunds received, so that either a nil or very small figure is included in those accounts. This is not acceptable; clear and precise instructions are included in the Red Book and the quotations of these are set out in the following paragraphs:

Drugs and appliances: para 44.12
Rent and rates: para 51.36
Ancillary staff: para 52.21
Doctors in health centres: para 53.4

For the first time a suggestion has been made that accountants preparing accounts for GPs should certify these have been prepared on the lines illustrated above.

The generation of NHS income

As we have seen, ensuring the maximum level of profitability of the practice is one of the prime duties of a successful practice manager. She must be prepared, either herself or by suitable delegation, to ensure that:

1   the doctors are available to perform required levels of work for which the practice will receive payment;
2   a charge is made for such work, either NHS or private; and
3   payment is received for the work done within a reasonable period.

Let us now look at the main types of income which the practice can reasonably expect to receive from NHS sources and the means by which these are paid. The details of the 1990 Contract include:

Practice allowances

The full Basic Practice Allowance (BPA) is dependent upon a number of factors applying:

1   that the GP is a principal in his practice;
2   that the practice has an average of at least 1600 patients on each partner's list, otherwise a reduced allowance will be paid, but not to partners with less than 400 patients unless in an 'inducement' area;
3   in a partnership, he receives not less than one-third of the remuneration of the highest paid partner (there are variations for part-time partners); and
4   the GP works at least 26 hours per week on surgeries, visits, etc.

Proportionately lower rates of BPA will be paid in respect of part-time GPs and job-sharers.

Postgraduate Education Allowance

GPs have to submit evidence to their FHSA or Health Board of having attended an average of five days a year over the past five years. This will be phased in over the first five years. Courses are approved by Regional Advisers and there must be at least two under each of the headings:

Health promotion
Disease management
Service management

From 1 April 1991 following discrepancies between different regions in England, the Department of Health ruled that six hours would be equivalent to one day and there would be no half hours. There will now be no claim for expenses as these are included in the allowance. This new allowance replaces the vocational and postgraduate training allowance.

Seniority payments

These are paid in respect of years spent in practice:

First stage: registered 11 years: principal 7 years
Second stage: registered 18 years: principal 14 years
Third stage: registered 25 years: principal 21 years.

Capitation fees

This is a larger proportion of total income—around 60%—than previously. Higher fees are paid for the elderly. GPs are expected to offer patients over 75 at least one home visit annually and an assessment, for this an enhanced capitation fee is paid.

This forms an important part of income and it will be necessary to ensure that payment is received each quarter for patients who move into this age group.

Registration fees. A new capitation fee is paid for all patients over five years newly registering with a practice upon which certain procedures are carried out. These have to be done within three months of the patient joining the practice and payment will be made at the end of each quarter. It is essential to have a system for ensuring an appointment for all new registrations as soon as possible and within the same quarter if possible.

Childhood surveillance fees. GPs who are suitably trained and who are on the Child Surveillance List maintained by the FHSA are paid a special capitation fee for each child registered. GPs on the list will be able to offer the service to patients registered with their partners as well. Payments are made quarterly.

Item-of-service fees

It is upon the success or otherwise of claiming for fees of this nature that the financial success or failure of a practice will usually lie. In the case of the extreme example of two practices quoted earlier a major factor on the disparity in their incomes under the old scheme was due to their efficiency in claiming these fees. Whilst item-of-service fees will be a slightly smaller proportion of total income in the future nevertheless it will still be essential to maximize income in this way.

Night visit fees. A higher fee, three times larger, is paid if the night visit is made by a doctor from the patient's own practice or from a small, non-commercial rota of up to ten GPs. These fees can be claimed for visits carried out between the hours of 10 p.m. and 8 a.m.

Target payments

Childhood immunizations. There are two target levels, 70% and 90%, representing *average* cover across the three groups (i) diphtheria, tetanus and polio, (ii) whooping cough, (iii) mumps, measles and rubella. Target date is the first day of a quarter. All complete courses count towards coverage level wherever and by whomsoever they were done but the GP will only be paid for those he had done. So, if the GP had administered 70% of the course and the target reached was 90%, the payment would be $7/9$ of the maximum payment. The top level is paid at three times the rate of the lower level. The message is that the more immunizations done within the practice the greater the income and if top levels are secured it could result in about an extra £2000 p.a. per doctor to the practice. The same rules will apply for preschool boosters for children under five years.

Cervical cytology. There are two target levels of 50% or 80% of women between 25 and 64 who have had an adequate smear in the previous five and a half years by the first day of the quarter. The smear test may be done anywhere and women who have had a total hysterectomy will be excluded. The same rule applies that if the practice achieves the 80% level and half the smears were done in the practice, $5/8$ of the top level will be paid.

Sessional fees

Health promotion. A new fee is paid for health promotion clinics run within the practice relating to 'well person', diabetes, heart disease, anti-smoking, alcohol control, diet and stress management. With FHSA approval it is possible that other clinics may attract a sessional fee.

Minor surgery. A payment can be received for approved surgical procedures carried out. An average of five a month (up to 15 a quarter) will obtain the maximum payment.

Medical students. An allowance is paid to practices that have students to acknowledge the additional time spent.

Please ensure that for all of these payments the practice receives monthly payments on account. For the two intermediate months (say, January and February in the March quarter) a payment on account should be made at the end of each of those months, representing roughly one-third of the standing fees and allowances. These payments on account will then be shown as deductions on the subsequent quarterly statements.

Other NHS income

In many practices, income is derived from NHS sources outside the main fees and allowances paid by the FHSA. Some of this additional income is likely to take the form of salaries and remuneration from local hospitals or other NHS institutions. In a partnership care must be taken to ensure that these are properly treated and that the allocation of such income between the partners is in accordance both with their wishes and with the provisions of the partnership deed.

One major problem which derives from this source of income is the deductions which may well be taken before the net fees are received. These deductions are likely to take the form of superannuation, income tax and probably national insurance. The practice accountant should be consulted as to exactly how these are to be charged both to the partners in whose name the positions are held, and through the partnership accounts so as to ensure fairness and equity between the partners. These problems do not arise in the case of sole practitioners, the income being wholly that of the GP.

Non-NHS income

GPs are not restricted to earning their income from NHS sources and frequently they will go outside the NHS to earn a proportion of their income. In some cases this can be a relatively high proportion, particularly in 'police' practices and those living in an area which naturally attracts a high incidence of private patients.

In some practices a high source of earnings can result from retainers and annual fees paid by nursing homes, schools and commercial organizations for one or some of the partners acting as medical officer. It is wise to negotiate a realistic fee for this before the work is taken on and to have a suitable contract drawn up.

The typical practice, however, will receive a fairly steady source of income from insurance examinations and reports; cremation fees and sundry certificate money. You will see in the section on petty cash exactly how this money is to be dealt with but care must be taken to see that it is properly recorded in the books of the practice, both to ensure again that each partner receives his proper share of the income but also so that it does not give rise to an enquiry into fees not returned for tax purposes.

The allocation of this income in medical partnerships can frequently be a problem. It is usually advisable to have a rule that all income from medical sources, of whatever type, is to be aggregated with the partnership income and divided between the partners in agreed ratios. It is a ready-made source of friction between partners where some doctors retain part of their earnings, with their partners frequently feeling aggrieved at this not being put in the partnership pool.

Dispensing practices

In some cases practices will have the right to dispense drugs to patients on their lists. This is normally restricted to patients who live more than a mile from a chemist's shop. The doctors who are able to do dispensing work of this nature have a steady source of additional income, the dispensing fees being paid out in accordance with scales in force from time to time. A practice of this nature will probably employ a qualified dispenser who can deal with the detailed work on the dispensing of drugs. They will make returns to the FHSA from time to time; the prescriptions will be priced and a refund will ultimately be made to the partnership for the cost of those drugs, plus the dispensing fee.

It is common for such refunds to be made two or even three months in arrears. However, in order to obtain maximum discount, it is probably necessary to pay the wholesale chemist for supplying drugs at least monthly, so that the practice will need to have a fair measure of working capital in order to finance the stock of drugs which must be held at any given time.

Refunds

The practice will receive refunds in respect of rent (if it is a rented surgery), rates of various descriptions, ancillary staff and staff national insurance contributions. These recovery rates may be affected by cash limiting procedures imposed by the FHSA.

Where refunds of rates are claimed, care must again be taken to ensure that all refunds of such items as sewerage and water rates, drainage rates in certain areas and the like are also claimed. In some cases it will be possible to claim a refund of local authority refuse collection charges as well for the disposal of 'sharps'. In some urban areas, it may be possible to claim a refund of car parking contract charges paid to local authorities. Some practices lose thousands of pounds a year by not submitting these claims in a regular and efficient manner.

In addition to this and to the refunds of drugs described above, training practices must claim a refund of their trainee's salaries. Although not strictly speaking a refund, if doctors are away for reasons of sickness or on maternity leave, an allowance might be claimed in certain circumstances, which is intended to cover the cost of employing a locum.

Care must be taken to see that staff-related refunds (salaries, national insurance, training costs) are claimed at quarterly intervals and that payments on account for the two intermediate months are obtained. Although not actually generating additional income, this will greatly benefit the cash flow of the practice.

Managers should be aware of the new cash-limiting controls imposed by some FHSAs and how these will operate in respect of their particular practice. These controls may vary between areas. The controls may be particularly relevant, for example, ancillary staff refunds. Some FHSAs have already declined to refund in respect of new, or some cases, replacement staff.

Leave advances

A great help to the cash flow of both the practice and the individual doctors is the claiming of the leave advance. This is 20% of the Basic Practice Allowance and should be claimed by submission of Form FP75 to the FHSA by 15 April each year.

Internal control questionnaire for medical practices

1 General accounting organization

(a) Are the accounting records maintained up-to-date and balanced monthly?

(b) Do the partners appear to take a direct and active interest in the financial affairs of the practice?

(c) Are there any systems of periodic financial reports or budgetary control?

(d) Are the personal funds and financial transactions of the partners completely segregated from the partnership?

2 Receipts

(a) Is the mail opened by the partners?

(b) Are sundry cash receipts separately recorded?

(c) Is money received banked intact?

3   Payments

(a)   Are all payments made by cheque?
(b)   Can cheques be signed only by the partners?
(c)   Are cheques signed only when complete (i.e. not blank)?
(d)   Is supporting documentation approved and cancelled by the partners when payment is made?
(e)   Is supporting documentation properly filed, consecutively numbered and cross-referenced to the cash book?
(f)   Are spoiled cheques retained?
(g)   Are payments not made by cheque (e.g. standing orders) authorized only by the partners?
(h)   Do the partners review the bank reconciliations?
(i)   Is petty cash maintained on an imprest system?

4   Fees and debtors (for private patients)

(a)   Are fee notes pre-numbered and all accounted for?
(b)   Is a list of unpaid fees regularly reviewed by the partners?
(c)   Are reminders sent to patients in respect of overdue fees?

5   Drawings

(a)   Are partners' drawings paid regularly (e.g. monthly)?
(b)   Do the calculations for regular drawings take account of tax reserves, disparities in allowances, etc.?
(c)   Are the amounts of regular drawings periodically reviewed during the year in the light of practice income and any changes in profit sharing ratios?
(d)   Are Class 2 National Insurance Contributions paid regularly by the partnership and debited to the partners' current accounts?

6   Wages and salaries

(a)   Are employees taken on or dismissed only by the partners?
(b)   Are references obtained in respect of new employees?
(c)   Are PAYE and National Insurance deductions paid over monthly to the Collector of Taxes?

7   Fixed assets

(a)   Are detailed records maintained of the assets owned by the practice?
(b)   Are the partners aware of which assets are owned by the practice and which are owned by the individual partners?
(c)   Are disposals and scrapping of assets authorized only by the partners?

8   Stock (for dispensing practices)

(a)   Are continuous stock records maintained?

(b)   Is stock physically counted periodically and reconciled to the stock records and dangerous drugs book?

Control of outgoings

We have had a look at means by which income can be maximized. However, this is by no means the full story. In order to achieve maximum profitability, some control must also be kept on outgoings and it is only by some sound method of budgeting and constant cost control that the practice is run in as economic a manner as possible.

One essential feature of the control of costs is the drawing up of a proper expenditure budget, it is suggested by the practice manager and agreed by the partners before the commencement of each financial year. For this it is necessary to know the date to which the partnership's annual accounts are prepared. This will normally be one of the conventional quarter days, i.e. 31 March, 30 June, 30 September or 31 December. Whichever date is used, the budget should be formulated and agreed as soon as possible beforehand. It may be that, following the completion of the practice accounts by the accountant, which at its earliest cannot for practical reasons take place at less than a few months after the end of each financial year, the budget will need to be revised, but a close monthly check should be kept on expenditure and if necessary checks and economies instituted.

It may be that there are exceptional items which cannot be controlled; for instance, a partner may be required to take sickness or maternity leave which involves the partnership in additional locum expenses. There may be unforeseen repairs required to the building or an exceptional increase in telephone or heating charges, but it is normally possible to build in some leeway in the budget to cater for these.

Table 11.1 illustrates a typical but simplified expenditure budget for a training practice of five partners. This shows the annual budgeted cost; the monthly actual and cumulative costs for the first two months of the year, October and November 1991 and how it is possible to make a running check of expenses by this means.

Before doing this it is important to specify which items of expenditure are to be paid out of the partnership account and which are to be borne by the individual partners personally. A number of items of expenditure may well be paid by either of these means, depending on partnership policy. This should be clearly specified beforehand and set out in precise terms in the partnership deed so as to leave no room for misinterpretation. Such items could well be:

Partners' car expenses
Private telephone charges

Spouses' salaries, pensions, etc.
Medical subscriptions
Private accountancy fees

If these are to be borne individually by the partners they should not be included as items of expenditure in any practice budget.

If this applies, such items should ideally not be paid out of partnership funds. Although honour can be satisfied by charging these to the partners' current accounts, as merely an extra item of drawing, nevertheless this is likely to give rise to big inequalities between the partners at the end of each year, which must be balanced annually. It is therefore advised that such personal items of expenditure be paid by the partners out of their own bank accounts and not out of partnership funds.

Table 11.1 Expenditure budget.

Control Sheet: Year to 31 September 1991

	Annual budget cost (£)	October 1991		November 1991	
		Actual (£)	To date (£)	Actual (£)	To date (cumulative) (£)
Drugs and appliances	2000	–	–	100	100
Locum fees	3000	–	–	–	–
Deputizing	1000	50	50	50	100
Equipment hire	1500	200	200	150	350
NHS levies	500	–	–	–	–
Training costs	600	50	50	30	80
Books and journals	100	–	–	20	20
Staff salaries (inc. NIC)	30 000	2500	2500	2350	4850
Trainees' salaries	15 000	1250	1250	1250	2500
Staff welfare	1000	100	100	50	150
Recruitment costs	500	–	–	80	80
Rates and water	5300	400	400	400	800
Light and heat	1500	–	–	150	150
Repairs and renewals	2000	500	500	100	600
Insurance premiums	800	–	–	200	200
Cleaning and laundry	2000	200	200	200	400
Garden expenses	500	50	50	20	70
Printing, stationery and postage	1800	500	500	200	700
Telephone	4800	500	500	200	700
Accountancy	4200	–	–	–	–
Bank charges	200	–	–	100	100
Legal charges	200	–	–	100	100
Sundry expenses	1500	200	200	100	300
TOTAL BUDGETED COSTS	80 000	6500	6500	5850	12 350

Basic bookkeeping and accounts

General practice, is a business; probably a very big business. Even a small practice will have a turnover running into six figures.

Were this a conventional business enterprise, it would likely as not employ skilled accounting staff to deal with its affairs and the problem of inadequate records would not apply. Doctors, however, are notoriously bad both at keeping their own personal records and those of their practices or partnerships.

Most doctors have had no financial training whatever. Yet in entering general practice they might well find themselves, within a relatively short period, equity partners in a medium-sized business enterprise, having to participate in any number of far-reaching decisions affecting the finances of themselves, their partners and their staff; employment and staffing; budgeting and controls; taxation, insurance, banking and investment.

It need hardly be said that such decisions as have to be taken regularly in all medical practices are virtually impossible without access to proper, well-maintained and comprehensive accounting records. Hopefully those records will be kept, or at the very least supervised, by a competent practice manager and they will form the basis of the practice's financial reporting facility. No true business decisions can be made without them.

One is frequently asked why records of this nature should be kept; why it could not all by kept by an accountant. The prime reasons for keeping such bookkeeping records are:

1 to identify items of income and to highlight means by which this can be maximized;
2 conversely, to keep a close watch on expenditure and through successful budgeting control costs economize;
3 by means of the above, to maximize profits and hence the income of the partners;
4 the partnership deed may well include a clause to the effect that 'proper bookkeeping records shall be kept';
5 records will be available in the event of enquiry by the Inland Revenue into the practice's affairs; and
6 a possible saving in accounting fees.

It is sometimes found that outside accountants keep the books of the practice but this will almost certainly cost the partners a great deal of money. Accountants' time is expensive and it is wholly uneconomic to have a professional person dealing with routine bookkeeping records of this nature.

One advantage not possessed by any other business, as we have seen, is the facility to recover some or all of the costs of employing ancillary staff and their national insurance contributions. This can be extended to include clerical staff such as bookkeepers and it obviously makes financial sense to employ one's own staff for this purpose rather than to use an accountant, whose fees will not only be expensive but will certainly not be recoverable, either wholly or partly from the FHSA, as well as including a 17½% VAT charge.

Firstly let us look briefly at the type of bookkeeping records which should be kept.

Petty cash

The basic record for all cash transactions is the petty cash book, probably with the actual cash on hand on any given date being maintained in one or two petty cash boxes specifically used for that purpose. The maintenance of an efficient and well-regulated system of petty cash control and recording is an integral part of the practice's bookkeeping arrangements.

What exactly is meant by petty cash? It does of course mean coin of the realm and bank notes, either received by the practice from patients as fee income or available in the form of a float, from which sundry cash disbursements can be made. These two aspects of petty cash in the average general practice should be kept entirely distinct.

It cannot be too strongly emphasized that any fees received in cash, of whatever nature, for certificates, sundry other fees, and especially cremation fees should be properly accounted for and paid into the practice bank account without deduction.

The notion is incorrect (but nevertheless it persists) that these fees are in some way 'perks' which need not be accounted for and which the doctor is entitled to put into his pocket without paying tax on. Nothing could be further from the truth; these are the income from his profession and it is essential that they are fully accounted for, both for accountancy and taxation purposes.

There are some doctors who have had a rude shock recently by finding that, for instance, cremation fees have been traced by the Inspector of Taxes and that they are asked to pay tax upon them, for several years in arrears.

Cash receipts of this nature should always be collected together separately and paid to the practice bank periodically. Many practices retain such cash on hand in a separate tin for a period of, say, a week or a fortnight, or perhaps upon reaching a previously agreed sum.

A great deal will depend on the circumstances of the practice and the volume of fees received, but a policy once established should be strictly adhered to.

It is also recommended that a separate book (*see* Fig. 11.1) be kept to record these sundry fees received, not only as a routine record but to enable the practice manager to check whether any given fee has been received. This could have a separate column for recording receipts of a non-fee nature and it is also suggested that a separate column be maintained for recording

	SUNDRY CASH RECEIPTS – MAY 1989		Fees		Other		
May 1	Mr Brown – fee		2	50			
	Mr Smith – examination		5	85			
	Mrs Green – private patient		7	50			
2	Mr Jones – certificate			50			
	Staff telephone refund				3	75	
	Mrs Harrison – private patient		5	25			
	XYZ Insurance Co. – examination		7	00			
4	Dr Williams – Locum fee		10	00			
		£	38	60	3	75	
	Paid to bank 5/5/1989	£	42	35			

Figure 11.1 A specimen page from a sundry cash receipts book.

cremation fees. The actual cash should be collected in a separate cash tin retained for this purpose only, which is cleared fully when the periodic bankings are made.

Once again, it cannot be emphasized too strongly that the mixing of sundry cash receipts of this nature, with cash retained for payment of sundry petty cash items, should be discouraged. For payments such as this, a separate cheque should be drawn from the bank periodically, based upon an average weekly or monthly expenditure and replenished from time to time by a cashed cheque drawn on the practice bank account. This should also be kept in a separate cash tin maintained for payment purposes. Doctors and staff requiring cash for any purpose should be asked to complete either a petty cash voucher or to submit a receipt. Once made, all such payments should be regularly and systematically recorded in a petty cash book used only for this purpose. The payments petty cash book should ideally be in the form of an analysis book, which should be regularly added up and balanced and reconciled with the cash held in the tin.

A specimen page from a typical payments petty cash book is shown (Fig. 11.2).

Receipts, in the form of cash withdrawn from the bank, should be shown on the left-hand (or debit) side. Payments should be shown on the right-hand (or credit) side, being entered once in the payments (or 'total') column and again in the most appropriate analysis column.

RECEIPTS	PAYMENTS	Postage	Stationery	Partners' National Insurance	Cleaning	Repairs	Locum fees	Refreshments	Sundries	
32 97										
	21 95	11 95		10 −						
	5 75		5 75							
	4 50				4 50					
40 −										
	5 50				5 50					
	1 25								1 25	
	6 80							6 80		
	10 −						10 −			
	4 75					4 75				
	23 60	10 −		13 60						
	2 65		2 65							
	5 25							5 25		
50 −										
	1 50								1 50	
	4 50								4 50	
	6 50				6 50					
122 97	104 50									
		21 95	8 40	23 60	16 50	4 75	10 −	12 05	7 25	
	18 47									
£ 122 97	122 97									

A few days' entries in a typical cash book. A narration giving details of each entry would normally be shown on the left-hand side.

Figure 11.2

The headings of the various analysis columns depend largely on the circumstances of the particular practice, but again they should be totalled periodically and, if the entries have been made correctly, the sum of the total of the various analysis columns should equal that of the payments (or total column). These can all be totalled monthly and a balance carried forward to the start of the following month. A test balance can be taken at any time, merely by finding the difference between the running totals of the receipts and payments columns. This should then be compared with the cash held in the tin and any difference investigated.

Differences in the cash held may well occur, more often than not for entirely innocent reasons; a payment might have been omitted from the petty cash book or an incorrect entry made. However, the majority of funds passing through the practice will represent payments into and withdrawals from, the practice bank account. We now look at how this should be properly written up and reconciled (*see* Fig. 11.3, opposite).

1990		Details	TOTAL	NHS	Appointments	Insurance Exams, etc	Sundry fees	Other receipts
Jan 1	Balance bt/forward		2,653 94					
	H.Smith – fee	5 –					5 –	2653 94
	ABC Insurance Co.	9 –				9 –		
	DEF Insurance Co.	9 –				9 –		
3	GHI Insurance Co.	9 –				9 –		
	JKL Insurance Co.	9 50				9 50		
	Income tax repaid	127 85						127 85
	County College	350 –			350 –			
5	MNO Insurance Co.	9 50				9 50		
	Private certificate	2 –					2 –	
7	B.J.Funeral–Crem. fee	16 50	547 35				16 50	
11	PQR Insurance Co.	9 50				9 50		
	STU Insurance Co.	9 –				9 –		
13	Loamshire County Council	15 –					15 –	
	Mr Jones – fee	20 –					20 –	
14	Mr Brown – fee	25 –					25 –	
	Mr Williams – fee	30 –					30 –	
	XYZ Nursing Home	500 –			500 –			
17	ABC Insurance Co.	9 50				9 50		
	DEF Insurance Co.	9 –				9 –		
	Mr White	20 –					20 –	
18	Loamshire FHSA Rent & Rates		2,350 –	2,350 –				
20	GHI Insurance Co.	9 50				9 50		
	Mrs Green	35 –					35 –	
22	Loamshire Hospital Clinical Assistant	108 96			108 96			
23	JKL Insurance Co.	9 50	809 96			9 50		
24	Loamshire FHSA							
	Trainee refund		3,647 94	3,647 94				
	JKL Insurance Co.	9 50				9 50		
25	ABC Insurance Co.	9 50				9 50		
	Mr Black	56 –					56 –	
	Mr Blue	25 –					25 –	
28	Sundry cash takings	55 –					55 –	
	cremation fee	16 50	171 50				16 50	
31	Loamshire FHSA							
	Monthly advance		7,250 –	7,250 –				
	Ancillary staff		1,300 –	1,300 –				
		£	18,724 69	14,547 94	958 96	121 –	321 –	3781 79

1990		Cheque No.	Sub No.	TOTAL	Salaries	Drugs & instruments	Trainee payments	Locum fees	Rent and rates	Lighting & Heating	Cleaning	Telephone	Petty Cash	Repairs & rentals	Partners drawings	Tax reserve transfers	Sundries
Jan 1	Dr Jones: locum	635 46	1	100 –				100 –									
	Transfer	S.O.															
	Building Society			1,200												1,200 –	
2	Fire Insurance	47	2	85 76													85 76
3	Accountancy fees	48	3	2,575 –													2,575 –
	PAYE/NIC: Month 9	49	4	897 40	651 10		246 30										
4	Smart Drug Company	50	5	35 65		35 65											
	Electricity Board	51	6	152 75						152 75							
	Mrs Jones: cleaner	52		20 –							20 –						
6	Petty cash	53		50 –									50 –				
	Water Board	54	7	65 35					65 35								
9	Surgery rent	55	8	1,750 –					1,750 –								
	Gas Board	56	9	97 50						97 50							
11	Post Office: Telephone	57		267 45								267 45					
	Mr Brown: Plumb. repair	58		25 –										25 –			
	ZYX Instrument Co.	59		15 50		15 50											
15	Dr Jones: locum	60		150 –				150 –									
22	Cleaning materials	61		27 50							27 50						
	Coffee	62		10 75													10 75
24	Legal charges	63		250 –													250 –
25	Petty cash	64		50 –									50 –				
31	Mrs V Wiliams	65		268 45	268 45												
	Mrs J Smith	66		139 54	139 54												
	Mrs B Jones	67		235 46	235 46												
	Mrs D Johnson	68		226 92	226 92												
	Mrs S Green	69		137 50	137 50												
	Mrs A Watson	70		197 45	197 45												
	Mrs M Robinson	71		226 45	226 45												
	Mrs L White	72		57 50							57 50						
	Dr N Hunt: trainee	73		858 75			858 75										
	Borough Council & rates	S.O.		357 50					357 50								
	Staff pension scheme	S.O.		500 –													500 –
	Dr Grace	S.O.		2,200 –											2,200 –		
	Dr Hobbs	S.O.		2,000 –											2,000 –		
	Dr Bradman	S.O.		1,950 –											1,950 –		
	Dr Hutton	S.O.		675 –											675 –		
				17,856 13	2,082 87	51 15	1,105 05	250 –	2,172 85	250 25	105 –	267 45	100 –	25 –	6,825 –	1,200 –	3,421 51
	Balance c/forward			868 56													
			£	18,724 69													

Figure 11.3 The GP's cashbook—recommended column headings.

> ## Box 11.2: Petty cash recording
>
> *Do*
>
> Keep the cash proceeds from fees separate from cash used for making payments.
>
> Record cash fee income and pay to the practice bank account regularly.
>
> Make petty cash payments from float withdrawn from the bank for that purpose.
>
> Record payments in an analysis cash book.
>
> Total columns for each month and balance.
>
> Reconcile balance regularly with cash held in box.
>
> Ensure that petty cash drawn from bank is identically shown in both the petty cash receipts and payments cash book.
>
> ### *Do not*
>
> Mix up proceeds for cash fees with sundry cash payments.
>
> Keep inadequate records.
>
> Fail to count the cash regularly and check with balance.

Systems of drawings

In all partnerships there must be a system of withdrawing funds from the practice account by the partners, so that income can be passed to their own accounts for personal use. Doctors, like all other sections of the community, have their personal living expenses to finance and there must be some regular and controlled means of transferring funds to them.

For employees, such as hospital doctors, GP trainees and consultants, this is not a problem. They are employees and their salary will be paid to them, normally at the end of each month, having undergone all necessary deductions. GPs however are not employees; as we have seen, they are self-employed individuals and as partners they all have a responsibility to each other. One of these is to ensure that funds passed to them from time to time are in keeping both with their profit-sharing ratios and all other known factors.

Unfortunately, incorrect terminology can often be used in such areas and it can, and frequently is, highly misleading where doctors refer to these monthly amounts paid to them as their 'salary'. This is not the case and the fact cannot be emphasized too strongly. Indeed, the word 'salary' in itself has all manner of unfortunate connotations in this context, not least being the manner in which the income is taxed, and it is better to avoid the term if at all possible.

It is no exaggeration to say that the periodic calculation of these partnership drawings is one of the financial procedures which regularly causes most difficulties to GPs in partnership. Many doctors feel that knowledge of their incomes is of such a confidential nature that it cannot be delegated to a member of their staff. These calculations are therefore, in many cases, done by one of the partners themselves. Fortunately, attitudes are changing and in an increasing number of cases, such drawings calculations in fact will be done by a responsible practice manager.

Rather different problems concern the single-handed practitioner. He has no partners to worry about and the money he earns is his own, subject of course to making prudent provisions for income tax and other matters. He may however be well advised to pass all his professional transactions through a separate practice bank account and to transfer monthly such sums as can reasonably be set aside into his private bank account for his own use.

Drawings calculations should be done correctly, if partners are to avoid feeling they are receiving more or less than their proper entitlement, and in order to avoid disparities in their current accounts at the end of each financial year.

Whether drawings have been properly calculated or not will become evident when the annual partnership accounts are prepared and any differences in the current accounts of the partners will then become apparent. Steps should be taken to see that any continuing errors do not recur and that those balances are adjusted by subsequent and 'one-off' adjustments to drawings.

There are probably as many different systems of drawings by partners are there are fingers on one's hands. Whatever system is used, it is essential that it is operated properly. The simplest system of all, of course, would be in a two-man partnership sharing profits equally, so that both doctors could withdraw identical amounts. In practice, that is likely to be the exception rather than the rule. In virtually all cases, complex adjustments will be made for differing rates of seniority awards and the like; superannuation payments; added years contributions; loan interest charges; national insurance; repayments of leave advance, and other items.

The system which is perhaps most widely used in partnerships is the 'month-end' or 'quarter-end' system, under which partners are paid out at the end of each month, adjustments being made quarterly to take into consideration the factors mentioned above. Whilst it is acceptable that payments at the end of the two intermediate months may be made in partnership ratios, the full measure of adjustments must be made at the end of the quarter and this can perhaps best be illustrated by the example shown in Fig. 11.4. This shows a four-doctor partnership; Drs A, B, C and D, the three senior partners having a share of 28% and a new partner, Dr D, with a share of 16%. Drs A and B are both paying for added-years (A); all the partners are paying leave advances (B); whilst Dr D has a loan from the GP Finance Corporation (C). Drs A, B and C have seniority awards at varying rates (D) and Dr D is entitled to a vocational training allowance (E). The figures shown are for illustration purposes only and it should not be assumed that these will apply to partnerships in practice.

Calculation of quarterly drawings: October 1990.

Drs A, B, C and D	Total £		Dr A 28%		Dr B 28%		Dr C 28%		Dr D 16%	
Balance in partnership bank account (F)	13 000									
Less:										
retain on hand (G)	4 500	8 500								
For distribution (H)										
Add: Deductions:										
Superannuation	540									
Added years (A)	120									
Leave advance (B)	1 200									
GPFC loan (C)	125									
Monthly on account	10 000	11 985								
		20 485								
Less:										
Additions to income:										
Seniority (D)	2 400									
VTA (E)	400									
PGTA	–	2 800								
For allocation (in partnership) ratios (i)		17 685		4 952		4 952		4 952		2 829
Add:										
Seniority (D)	2 400		1 000		1 000		400		–	
VTA (E)	400		–		–		–		400	
PGTA	–	2 800	–	1 000	–	1 000	–	400	–	400
		20 485		5 952		5 952		5 352		3 229
Less:										
Superannuation	540		150		150		150		90	
Added years (A)	120		75		45		–		–	
Leave advance (B)	1 200		300		300		300		300	
GPFC loan (C)	125	1 985	–	525	–	495	–	450	125	515
		18 500		5 427		5 457		4 902		2 714
Monthly on account		10 000		2 800		2 800		2 800		1 600
Net withdrawals		8 500		2 627		2 657		2 102		1 114

Figure 11.4

In computing the total amount to be distributed, it is normal to find the balance available on the partnership bank account (F), either by reference to the bank statements at the end of the quarter or, more preferably and where adequate and accurate records are kept, by referring to the balance in hand as shown in the practice cash book. There should be retained from the amount the estimated expenditure to run the practice during the succeeding months (G) and the balance will then be available for distribution (H).

It should be remembered that at the same time as this distribution is made, certain deductions have been made from the quarterly FHSA remuneration and, similarly, certain additions will have been included (*see* Box 11.3). It is necessary to reverse these entries before arriving at the total allocation for the quarter (I) and then to allocate the proper amounts to each of the four partners.

Box 11.3: Details of likely items to be adjusted on periodic drawings calculations

Income
- Seniority awards
- Vocational training allowance
- Postgraduate training allowance
- Notional rent allowance (where to be distributed in different ratios to partnership shares)

Outgoings
- Superannuation contributions:Standard
- Added years: Unreduced lump sum
- National insurance contributions
- Repayment of leave advances
- GPFC (or other) loan repayments and interest
- Transfers to income tax reserve

It may also be that certain of the partners do not own the surgery premises and they will not be entitled to share in any notional rent allowances in respect of the building. A detailed examination of the quarterly FHSA statement should be made, in order to ensure that all items of this nature are taken into account. Care should also be taken to see that all the income to be distributed has been earned during a period when current profit-sharing ratios were in operation. In many cases, NHS income is paid substantially in arrears. It must be allocated to the period in which it was actually earned and where such items of income have been received during one quarter, these should be taken out of the normal quarterly calculation and divided separately, in appropriate ratios.

Equalized drawings systems

Many partnerships are now becoming aware of systems of equalized drawings, under which a full year's net income is estimated and divided into equal amounts for distribution to the partners. Provided that all proper adjustments have been made, this regular monthly withdrawal can be paid to the partner's personal bank accounts by standing order.

This system allows a partner to estimate his regular monthly income, for the purpose of his own personal family budget and also avoids the constant calculation and issue of monthly cheques. The system is illustrated in the example shown (Fig. 11.5), in the case of a four-doctor partnership, with varying rates of superannuation, seniority, added-years and other items. This calculation is normally made on a tax-year basis, so that a reserve (*see* p. 164) can be made for the annual partnership income tax liability.

The detailed preparation of such an equalized drawings system will normally be done by the partnership accountant, who should have the required detailed information available to him and who will be in a position to calculate the tax reserve to be operated during any given period.

National insurance contributions (NIC)

Sometimes called 'the hidden income tax' because, although it is calculated on a taxpayer's income, it receives relatively little publicity and changes made are not normally announced in each year's budget, NIC can account for a surprisingly large slice of an individual's income.

There are basically four separate classes of insurance, all of which the practice manager should be aware of, particularly the going rates in force at any particular time and the manner in which these are collected.

Class 1

Class 1 NIC is paid by deduction from an employee's wage or salary. It is calculated by means of contribution tables and paid over to the Inland Revenue by the employer each month together with the staff PAYE deductions. Some employees, notably GP trainees, are 'contracted out' of the NHS scheme, which means that they are part of an employers scheme and consequently pay less contributions.

Class 2

Class 2 contributions are normally paid by stamping a contribution card, by self-employed people, including GPs. There is a facility for payment by direct debit, either from the personal account of the doctor concerned or from a partnership account. Most practices prefer to pay Class 2 NIC by stamping a contribution card every few weeks, the stamps being purchased from the Post Office for that purpose. These contributions are the personal liability of the doctor concerned and are not an item of partnership expense. They should properly be charged to his current account along with his drawings.

Calculation of equalized drawings year 1991/92 (to March 1992)

	Total	Dr A (28%) £	Dr B (28%) £	Dr C (24%) £	Dr D (20%) £
Estimated partnership profits for year	90 000	25 200	25 200	21 600	18 000
Seniority awards	5 900	3 900	2 000	–	–
Vocational training allowance·	1 500	–	–	–	1 500
Total income (est) (1)	97 400	29 100	27 200	21 600	19 500
Deductions					
Superannuation (est)	5 600	1 600	1 500	1 300	1 200
Added years	1 300	800	300	200	–
On outside appts (est)	100	–	20	80	–
National insurance (est):					
Class I (appointments)	100	–	–	100	–
Class II (stamps)	960	240	240	240	240
Repayment of leave advance	4 824	1 206	1 206	1 206	1 206
Repayment of loans (GPFC)	1 300	–	–	500	800
	14 184	3 846	3 266	3 626	3 446
Income tax reserve					
1984/5	18 000	6 500	5 500	4 000	2 000
Total outgoings (2)	32 184	10 346	8 766	7 626	5 446
Net (1–2)	65 216	18 754	18 434	13 974	14 054
Monthly (÷ 12)	5 434	1 563	1 536	1 164	1 171
(but say) . . .	5 415	1 560	1 530	1 160	1 165

Figure 11.5

Class 3

Class 3 contributions are paid only by non-employed people. In most cases these are paid by those individuals who have taken early retirement and wish to preserve their pension rights which, for a man, will not apply until age 65.

Class 4

Class 4 contributions are paid on a band of income which changes from year to year. For the 1991/92 year, earnings falling within this band of income are assessed at 6.3% and the maximum amount which can be paid by any contributor is £803.25.

The practice manager is strongly advised to ensure that all doctors in the practice have a National Insurance record. New partners should be encouraged to approach their own DSS office with a view to obtaining a contribution card. If this is not done it can result in arrears of contributions being charged, possibly running into several hundreds or even thousands of pounds and this is best avoided if at all possible.

Rates of contributions for the 1991/92 years are set out in Appendix D.

The use of income tax reserve accounts

We have had a look at the manner in which drawings calculations are made and that these will take into account the practice's tax liabilities. Tax will normally be payable in two instalments on 1 January and 1 July. Many practices, for reasons of cash-flow benefit and security, prefer to set regular amounts aside in a separate deposit or building society account, from which these payments might be made as and when they fall due. Systems of this nature have two main advantages.

1   They avoid the drawing of large cheques by individual partners twice a year, often with fairly traumatic results on the individual's own finances.
2   They avoid the possibility of a retiring partner leaving a tax liability behind him, which may well fall on the continuing partners.

The time scale for the operation of such a reserve is important and to a great degree depends on the estimates of future liabilities being received as early as possible within each separate tax year.

Under the normal preceding year basis of assessment, a practice with a year-end on, say, June 30 will find that the profits earned in the year ending on that date will be assessable in the following tax year. In the case of a practice making up its accounts to 30 June 1990, the tax assessment based on those profits would be the tax year 1991/92. It would normally be possible for an accountant to make a reasonable estimate of the tax payable before the start of the actual year of assessment. With a 31 March year-end, however, it may well be May or June within the actual tax year that even a preliminary estimate can be prepared.

The reserve should be held physically separate from the main partnership funds, either in a building society or bank deposit account, the periodic interest being divided between the partners in proportion to their shares of the balance on hand. It should preferably be transferred by means of a monthly standing order from the main partnership bank account, on a tax year basis so that for, say, the 1991/92 year, 12 monthly transfers would be made, commencing at the end of April 1991 until March 1992.

A typical reserve is illustrated in the example (Fig. 11.6). This shows a four-doctor practice with an estimated liability for 1991/92 of £18 000. This could well have been calculated in, say, January or February 1991 and may require some amendment to take account of amended allowances and tax rates which have been introduced in the 1991 Budget. Interest will be credited to the various partners in proportions to their differential contributions.

Income tax reserve

	Annual tax liability 1989/90 £	Monthly reserve April 1989 – March 1989/90 £
Dr W	6 000	495
Dr X	5 000	410
Dr Y	4 750	390
Dr Z	2 250	185
	18 000	1 480

The monthly transfer can be slightly less than a 12th of the annual liability, due to interest which will be credited to the account.

Figure 11.6

The role of the accountant

The average practice will use many financial advisers during its normal operations. Some of these, such as the lawyer and the architect they may well see infrequently, the bank manager probably at rather more frequent intervals. But it will be the accountant who effectively will have overall control over the practice finances, to whom they will most closely relate and who will be in most ready contact with them. In practice this contact will frequently take place via the practice manager, who will be responsible for reporting to her doctors the recommendations of the accountant on numerous matters, including drawings, tax reserves, etc.

It is very important that the accountant should be one who has specialized in medical finance, hopefully for many years and has a number of GP clients from whom he can gather his experience and speciality. Many practices find difficulty in relating to an accountant who does not understand the strange ways of doctors' finances and express constant dissatisfaction.

The relationship between the doctor, the practice manager and the accountant should properly be one of confidence and even friendship.

All too often and unfortunately it degenerates, possibly through misunderstandings on both sides, to mutual resentment and often to a parting of the ways. Many practices, through lack of knowledge of the accountant's function, find it difficult to judge whether he is doing his job properly and this guideline could well assist in consolidating their views. In judging potential candidates for the practice accountant, a number of criteria should be borne in mind.

Is he a specialist?

Does he have a copy of the Red Book and is he conversant with topics of medical finance, such as cost-rent schemes, doctors superannuation, practice allowances and numerous other items?

Efficiency

Are letters answered promptly and telephone calls returned? Are the accounts delivered within a relatively brief period; are tax, pension queries, etc. dealt with expeditiously?

Fee levels

This is discussed in more detail below but generally speaking the level of fees charged should not be a major item in deciding who will be the practice accountant. Of far more importance is whether he is capable, and demonstrates his ability to do an efficient and specialist job for the practice.

Proximity

Many practices feel they need an accountant working virtually from the next street. With modern methods of communication this is by no means as necessary as it might have been in the past. The times when the practice manager or doctors will need to consult their accountant personally in the same office will usually be few and far between and most accountants will arrange in any event to visit the practice at least once or twice yearly for a full discussion.

Fees

All accountants calculate their fees by means of an hourly charge which may vary from firm to firm but which will reflect the seniority, experience and aptitude of the individual partner or staff member dealing with the work.

It follows that it is in the interest of the practice to minimize that work so much as is possible. For instance, a bookkeeping system on the lines illustrated on page 170 will almost certainly result in a lower level of fees than a system which is either non-existent, inadequately written up or inaccurately presented. Accountants' fees will include an addition of 17½% VAT, which is not part of the actual fee retained by the accountant but must be paid over by him to the Inland Revenue. Nevertheless, as doctors are unable to register for VAT it is effectively an additional cost to their practice.

The judgement of accounting fees is extremely difficult and dependent on numerous factors, but as a very rough and general guideline, fee levels, which exclude personal work for the individual partners, should probably fall within the range of 1% to 2% of gross practice income. If they exceed that level, the practice will be quite reasonable in expecting justification to be supplied. On the other hand, if these fall below those factors, there could be a possibility that the accountant is spending insufficient time on the practice affairs, or using inexperienced staff. A practice with a gross turnover, including fee income and refunds, of £300 000 could probably expect therefore an annual charge, at current fee levels, of not less than £3000 inclusive of VAT, but exclusive of work done on the partners' personal affairs.

Duties

The accountant's duties will be many and varied. Basically he will prepare the practice accounts, having these agreed both by the partners and by the Inland Revenue for tax purposes. In addition he should be prepared to give additional advice on such matters as surgery development; calculation of tax reserves and drawings; provide statistical and management information concerning the practice income, expenditure and profits; advise the doctors on their pension arrangements; deal with personal tax affairs, claiming of practice expenses and numerous other items. It follows that he should be familiar with the Red Book and be able to interpret this as required.

Upon engagement an accountant should always be asked to give a quotation of his fees and should be expected to stick by this unless there are any factors of which he was not aware at the time it was made.

Surgery premises

One other aspect in which the finance of medical practices is significantly different from that of other businesses is that concerning the means by which surgery premises are financed.

Basically, for doctors practising from surgeries predominantly for the use of NHS patients, either a refund of rental payments is made, in the case of doctors practising from rented surgeries or, in the case of surgeries owned by the partners an allowance, in the form of either a notional or cost-rent allowance, will be paid to the practice.

Rented surgeries

These may fall under a number of different headings. Firstly, a fairly basic case of a surgery rented from a third-party landlord, to whom a rent is paid. It will be necessary for the rent receipt to be submitted to the FHSA after payment and this should be done as soon as possible. Provided that the whole of the surgery or building subject to the rent charge is allowable and falls under the qualifying rules, a full refund will be made.

Health centres

Many doctors practice from health centres and should ensure that the charge for rent and rates, which will not actually pass through the accounts of the practice, is ascertained. This should be handed to the accountant as he will be required to show it in the annual accounts as an item of expense and refund each year (*see* accounts in the next section, pp. 173 and 174 and para 53.45 of the Red Book).

Proportions of ownership

It may well be that the surgery is owned by not all the partners in the practice and indeed arrangements of this nature are extremely common, probably because some or all of the partners who may not have a full-time commitment, do not wish to become involved in property ownership.

It is important that this is established as it affects the allocation of the rent allowance and the cost of servicing any loans which have been taken out to buy or develop the property. It is important that this is understood, is shown clearly in the partnership deed and, if necessary, reflected in the drawings calculations.

Cost-rent schemes

Schemes of developing new, or adapting additional, surgery buildings under the cost-rent scheme are now extremely common and are an excellent means by which the partners in a practice can acquire a valuable interest in a commercial building without any appreciable capital outlay.

Such schemes are extremely complex both in their initial organization and in their subsequent administration. This should not be embarked upon without lengthy detailed and knowledgeable advice from professional people: an architect, a solicitor and an accountant, experienced in this type of work. This should be done in partnership with your FHSA who has the last word in deciding what the rent allowance will be and the means by which it will be calculated.

A note of current building limits for cost-rent schemes is set out in Appendix B.

How to read a set of accounts

Starting on page 172 is a typical set of accounts which might be produced for a general practice partnership of five doctors. This is the type of accounts which should be delivered to the partners by the practice accountant each year, as soon as possible after the accounting year-end. The accounts themselves have been designed to take into account several aspects which are unique to general practice and it is important that these and other points are understood in reading the accounts.

1 *Comparative figures:* On pages 172–174, which set out the profit, income and expenditure of the practice, it will be seen that the column on the right-hand side gives comparatives with the previous year's figures. These should always be shown in a set of accounts to give an easy comparison and so that trends in income and expenditure are apparent.

2 *Profit for the year:* Page 172 shows that the partnership during the year has realized a total profit of £168 228, an increase of 13.5% on the figure of £148 167 shown in the previous year. It is important that the concept of profit is understood; this is the means by which any business finances itself and, in the case of general practice, from which the partners earn their living.

3 *Split periods:* It will be seen from page 172 that the profits for the year have been divided into two sections. The profits realized were divided as to £75 354 in the first half-year and £87 474 in the second half-year. It may be thought that the profits should be divided equally over the two half-years but this is manifestly not the case. In general practice, profits are unlikely to be earned equally on a time apportionment basis and it would be quite wrong to show them as such in the accounts. It is equally important that this principle is understood as an incorrect allocation in this manner could well lead to partners suffering when the profits are divided between them in agreed ratios.

4   *Surgery income:* The left-hand column of page 172 shows that the surgery is owned by only three partners, Drs Black, White and Green. They own it equally and so have consequently been credited with one-third each of the net income accruing from their ownership.

5   *Income:* Page 173 sets out details of the income earned by the partnership during the year, both by way of NHS fees, various refunds and income from outside the National Health Service. Again, it is easy to obtain a comparison with the previous year.

6   *Payments:* Page 174 of the accounts shows similarly the payments made by the practice during the year, the allocation between the various profit-sharing periods and the manner in which the expenses have been divided.

7   Page 172 shows the partners who have been in the practice during the year and how they have been remunerated.

8   The balance sheet on page 175 sets out the financial position at any given date. It is normal practice for the accounts to be drawn up to the same date each year, in this case 31 March, and the balance sheet merely gives details of the assets and liabilities of the practice but, more importantly, the manner in which these have been contributed by the partners.

   In the case of this particular practice, being a surgery-owning partnership, there are shown property capital accounts, which represent the investment of three partners in the surgery premises. It will be seen that the total of those property capital accounts (£22 500) equals exactly the amount of the equity in the property shown in upper part of the balance sheet.

   Similarly, the investment of the partners in the fixed assets of the practice is represented by their capital accounts, whilst the net current assets are represented by the partners' current accounts. This concept of capital in medical partnerships is a complex point and one which it is necessary to understand fully for proper appreciation of GPs' partnership accounts.

9   It is common, in order to give an easy reading of the accounts, for a number of items in the balance sheet and elsewhere to be set out in notes to the accounts and these are set out on pages 176–178.

10 The partners' current accounts on page 179 are in effect their bank accounts with the practice. They give details of the profits earned by each partner; any seniority and similar awards which might be added to those profits, and the manner in which these have been paid out to the partners, in terms of drawings, superannuation, national insurance, income tax, etc.

   The final balances on those accounts must be equalized each year, usually by differential withdrawals by the partners, if fairness is to be obtained. Failure to operate this equalization procedure each year will almost certainly result in a 'snowball' effect over a number of years, with the disparity between the partners' current account balances increasing steadily until it reaches an unacceptable level.

11   Page 180 represents the drawings of the practice of the partners (*see* p. 158). Drawings are no more than the payments on account of the profits being earned by the partners. It is difficult for these to be calculated accurately during the year, which gives rise to the equalization procedure outlined above.

The practice manager should, in an enlightened and forward-looking practice, be made familiar with the practice accounts; in many partnerships a separate set of the accounts will be made available for her and she would be expected to discuss these with the partners. Certainly she should be invited to any meetings with the accountants when matters of a financial nature are being discussed.

Income and expenditure account, year ended 31.3.91.

	Surgery	Practice		1991	1990
		Period to 30 Sept 1989	Period from 1 Oct 1990		
	£	£	£	£	£
Income	32 800	157 292	176 569	366 661	320 258
Expenditure	27 400	81 938	89 095	198 433	172 091
	5 400	75 354	87 474		
Net profit for year				168 228	148 167
Allocation of profit					
Dr Black	1800	19 592	19 244	40 636	38 919
Dr White	1800	19 592	19 244	40 636	38 919
Dr Green	1800	19 592	19 244	40 636	38 919
Dr Patel	–	16 578	19 244	35 822	31 410
Dr Brown	–	–	10 498	10 498	–
	5400	75 354	87 474	168 228	148 167

Profits have been divided in the following ratios:		%	%
Dr Black	1/3	26	22
Dr White	1/3	26	22
Dr Green	1/3	26	22
Dr Patel	–	22	22
Dr Brown	–	–	12

Income

	Surgery	Practice					
		Period to 30 Sept 1990	Period from 1 Oct 1990	1991			1990
	£	£	£	£	£		£
National Health Service							
Capitation fees	–	46 952	47 492	94 444			91 250
Item-of-service fees	–	6876	8045	14 921			8057
Maternity fees	–	3851	4405	8256			7405
Practice allowances	–	19 795	27 768	47 563			44 873
				165 184			151 585
Trainee supervision grant	–	1670	1670	3340			3340
Rent allowance	32 000	–	–	32 000			32 000
Dispensing fees	–	2010	2165	4175			2760
					204 699		189 685
Refunds							
Health centre (per contra):							
Rent and rates	–	2000	2000	4000			3500
Ancillary staff	–	3165	3835	7000			6300
Rent: Main Surgery	–	16 000	16 000	32 000			32 000
Rates	–	1425	1425	2850			2500
Ancillary staff	–	8500	11 550	20 050			17 250
National insurance	–	2100	2317	4417			3800
Refuse collection	–	22	28	50			40
Trainee salaries	–	8000	8850	16 850			8500
Drugs	–	20 165	21 615	41 780			32 865
Locum fees (sickness)	–	–	400	400			–
					129 397		106 755
Appointments	–	8111	9754		17 865		12 768
Other fees							
Private patients	–	4000	4500	8500			6000
Insurance examinations etc	–	2000	2250	4250			3500
Cremations	–	100	150	250			200
Sundry	–	400	100	500			400
					13 500		10 100
Other income							
Building society interest	–	150	250	400			200
Rent for the clinic	800	–	–	800			750
					1200		950
Total income	32 800	157 292	176 569		366 661		320 258

Expenditure

	Surgery	Practice Period to 30 Sept 1990	Practice Period from 1 Oct 1990	1991	1991	1990
	£	£	£	£	£	£
Dispensing drugs						
Cost of drugs used	–	19 387	20 781		40 168	32 654
Practice expenses						
Drugs, instruments, etc	–	35	264	299		375
Locum fees	–	4700	1038	5738		6820
Relief service fees	–	1400	2300	3700		3000
Hire and maintenance of equipment	–	199	176	375		255
NHS levies	–	163	214	377		325
Practice replacements	–	125	–	125	–	75
Courses, conferences, books etc	–	85	–	85		50
					10 699	10 900
Staff expenses						
Salaries and ancillary staff	–	12 143	16 500	28 643		24 758
National insurance contributions	–	2100	2317	4417		3800
Salaries of trainee assistants	–	8000	8850	16 850		8500
					49 910	37 058
Surgery expenses						
Rent	–	16 000	16 000	32 000		32 000
Rates	–	1425	1425	2850		2500
Insurance	–	100	175	275		258
Lighting and heating	–	886	1478	2364		2158
Repairs and renewals	–	79	300	379		125
Cleaning	–	1138	1387	2525		1867
Garden expenses	–	205	53	258		235
					40 651	39 143
Health centre expenses						
Refunded per contra:						
Rent and rates	–	2000	2000	4000		3500
Ancillary staff (incl NIC)	–	4522	5478	10 000		9000
Running expenses	–	2450	2550	5000		4850
					19 000	17 350
Administration expenses						
Printing, stationery and postage	–	504	872	1376		1256
Telephone	–	1686	1900	3586		2555
Accountancy fees	–	1700	1550	3250		2975
Bank charges and interest	–	48	67	115		85
Sundries	–	220	549	769		715
Professional fees	–	–	233	233		–
					9329	7586
Financial expenses						
Surgery loan interest	27 400	–	–		27 400	27 400
Depreciation	–	638	638		1276	–
Total expenditure	27 400	81 938	89 095		198 433	172 091

Balance sheet for year ended 31 March 1991

	1991 £	1991 £	1990 £	1990 £
Surgery premises		22 500		10 000
Fixed assets		11 484		11 525
Funds held on income tax reserve		15 678		10 860
Current assets				
Stock of dispensing drugs	6351		5276	
Debtors	8386		6330	
Balance at building society	5750		2560	
Cash at bank: current account	4880		–	
Cash in hand	32		8	
	25 399		14 174	
Current liabilities				
Bank overdraft	12 404		5260	
Creditors	–		4875	
	12 404		10 135	
Net current assets		12 995		4039
		62 657		36 424
Partners' personal accounts				
Property capital accounts		22 500		10 000
Fixed asset capital accounts		11 484		11 525
Current accounts		12 995		4039
		46 979		25 564
Income tax reserve account		15 678		10 860
		62 657		36 424

Approved by the partners on   1991.

....
Dr W J Black

....
Dr S C White

....
Dr D M Green

....
Dr L F Patel

....
Dr R B Brown

Notes to the accounts year ended 31 March 1991

1. *Accounting policies*

    1.1 The income and expenditure account is prepared so as to reflect actual income earned, and expenditure incurred, during the year.

    1.2 The stock of dispensing drugs is valued at the lower of cost or net realizable value.

    1.3 Fixed assets other than surgery premises are written off over their estimated useful lives. The following rates of depreciation are applied to assets in use at the balance sheet date:

Fixtures and fittings	–	10% per annum
Medical and surgical equipment	–	10% per annum

2. *List sizes*

    Numbers of patients on the practice list, based upon capitation fees paid by the FHSA, during the period covered by the accounts were:

	Age:			
	To 64	65 – 74	75 & over	Total
1990: June	9821	978	628	11 427
September	9605	955	808	11 368
December	9750	980	705	11 435
1991: March	9807	995	667	11 469

3. *Health centre running costs*

    The practice occupies branch surgery accommodation in Brancaster Health Centre. Details shown in the accounts are as extracted from details supplied by the DHA.

    In accordance with standard recommendations, notional expenditure and refunds in connection with rent, rates and ancillary staff salaries have been shown on both sides of the account.

4. *Income from appointments*

		1991		1990	
		£	£	£	£
4.1	Hospital appointments				
	Dr Black	3175		3050	
	Dr Green	2065		1930	
			5240		4980
4.2	Other appointments				
	Brancaster Nursing Home	6500		5000	
	Brancaster Widgets Limited	3825		2788	
	Brancaster School	2300		–	
			12 625		7788
			17 865		12 768

Notes to the accounts *continued.*

5. *Surgery premises*

Cost

Branwell Surgery, Well Street, Brancaster
At 1 April 1990	275 000
Additions during year	–
At 31 March 1991	275 000

Fixed loans

National Branminster Bank PLC
At 1 April 1990	265 000
Repayments during year	12 500
At 31 March 1991	252 500

Net equity in surgery premises
At 31 March 1991	22 500
At 31 March 1990	10 000

6. *Fixed assets*

	Furniture and fittings £	Equipment £	Total £
Cost (or valuation)			
At 1 April 1990	15 072	6506	21 578
Additions during year	485	750	1235
	15 557	7256	22 813
Depreciation			
At 1 April 1990	5687	4366	10 053
Charge for year	987	289	1276
	6674	4655	11 329
Net book amounts			
At 31 March 1991	8883	2601	11 484
At 31 March 1991	9385	2140	11 525

7. *Property capital accounts*

	1991	1990
Dr Black	7500	3334
Dr White	7500	3333
Dr Green	7500	3333
	22 500	10 000

8. *Fixed asset capital accounts*

Dr Black	2527	2997
Dr White	2527	2997
Dr Green	2526	2996
Dr Patel	2526	2535
Dr Brown	1378	–
	11 484	11 525

Notes to the accounts *continued*.

		1991	1990
		£	£
9.	*Current accounts*		
	Dr Black	2850	1441
	Dr White	2968	1147
	Dr Green	3487	1173
	Dr Patel	1812	278
	Dr Brown	1878	–
		12 995	4039
10.	*Income tax reserve account*		
	Dr Black	4590	3415
	Dr White	4160	3150
	Dr Green	3501	2495
	Dr Patel	2613	1800
	Dr Brown	814	–
		15 678	10 860

11. *Dispensing practice: trading account*

	1991		1990	
	£	£	£	£
Cost of goods sold				
Stock at 1 April 1990		5276		4895
Purchases during year		41 243		33 035
		46 519		37 930
Less stock at 31 March 1991		6351		5276
		40 186		32 654
Proceeds				
Refunds (including VAT etc)	41 780		32 865	
Dispensing fees	4175		2760	
		45 955		35 625
Profit for year		5769		2971

Partners' current accounts year ended 31 March 1991

	Total		Dr Black		Dr White		Dr Green		Dr Patel		Dr Brown	
	£	£	£	£	£	£	£	£	£	£	£	£
Balances at 1 April 1990		4039		1441		1147		1173		278		–
Profit for the year	168 228		40 636		40 636		40 636		35 822		10 498	
Seniority awards	10 690		4730		2980		2980		–		–	
Vocational training allowances	2175		–		–				1450		725	
Postgraduate training allowance	655				–				655		–	
Leave advances	5872		1468		1468		1468		1468		–	
		187 620		46 834		45 084		45 084		39 395		11 223
		191 659		48 275		46 231		46 257		39 673		
Less: Partnership drawings												
Partners' monthly drawings	114 435		25 971		26 048		27 656		29 115		5645	
Transfers to income tax reserve account	33 400		9760		8850		7450		5560		1780	
Superannuation:												
Standard	7418		1884		1779		1779		1532		444	
Added years	3730		2165		1040		525		–		–	
National insurance contributiosn												
Class 1	472		286		186		–		–		–	
Class 2	878		195		195		195		195		98	
Leave advances repaid	5872		1468		1468		1468		1468		–	
	166 205		41 729		39 566		39 073		37 870		7967	
		25 454		6546		6665		7184		1803		3256
Transfers to/from retired partners' accounts												
Transfers to property capital accounts												
Surgery loan repayments	12 500		4166		4167		4167		–		–	
Transfers from fixed asset capital accounts												
Fixed asset additions	1235											
Less: depreciation	(1276)	(41)		(470)		(470)		(470)		(9)		(1378)
Balances at 31 March 1991	12 459	12 995	3696	2850	3697	2968	3697	3487		1812		1878

Partners' monthly drawings year ended 31 March 1991

		Total	Dr Black	Dr White	Dr Green	Dr Patel	Dr Brown
		£	£	£	£	£	£
1990:	April		1700	1700	1500	1400	–
	May		1700	1700	1500	1400	–
	June		1875	1800	1900	1600	–
	July		1800	1800	1600	1500	–
	August		1800	1800	1600	1500	–
			441	147	173	–	–
	September		2125	2070	1950	1850	–
	October		2000	2000	2000	2100	900
	November		2000	2000	2000	2100	900
	December		2175	2250	2500	2750	958
1991:	January		2500	2500	2500	2500	940
	February		2900	2900	2900	2500	940
	March		2955	3381	5533	7915	1007
		114 435	25 971	26 048	27 656	29 115	5645

The use of statistics in general practice

One advantage which medical practice has, which is not easily obtained for other businesses, is easy access to all manner of statistics which the doctors and practice manager can use to judge the profitability and efficiency of the practice. A few of these are set out below.

Expenditure levels

By the averaging process, and for superannuation purposes, the Department of Health considers that expenses of a medical practice are running at about 33.2% of gross income. This percentage is in fact unduly low; when one bears in mind that it takes into account any items paid personally by the partners, such as motor car expenses, houses, spouses' salaries, etc. It is to the doctors' advantage that this be maximized if at all possible, and this can only be done by the presentation of accounts which are drawn up in such a manner as to maximize the income and expenses of the practice.

Proportions of NHS income

The figures available at the present time, average proportions of NHS income received by a typical medical practice would be:

	To 31/3/90	From 1/4/90*
	%	%
Practice allowances	36	16
Capitation fees	47	60
Item-of-service fees	17	16
Target payments, etc.	–	8
	100	100

*Last available figures.

This is borne out by samples of accounts recently reviewed. Full figures for post-1990 GP Contract incomes are not yet available.

Item-of-service fees

A number of figures are available to give averages of item-of-service fees earned by medical practices in recent years. One of these (Fig. 11.7) gives the following as the average earnings of item-of-service fees per patient. This information is extremely valuable in attempting to evaluate the results of a practice.

Item-of-service fees—national averages

	England	Wales	Scotland	Northern Ireland
Night visits	39.0p	42.0p	45.9p	49.6p
Cervical cytology	17.9p	16.5p	13.4p	9.2p
Temporary residents	24.5p	34.5p	24.9p	11.7p
Contraceptive services	65.5p	56.5p	61.3p	42.5p
Emergency treatment etc.	2.5p	2.6p	5.3p	2.4p
Maternity medical services	105.0p	101.5p	96.6p	129.3p
Vaccinations/immunizations	60.6p	36.9p	48.3p	46.1p
Total average per patient	£3.15	£2.91	£2.96	£2.91

Calculated from figures supplied by health departments.

Figure 11.7

Financial information—and where to find it

The practice manager who wishes to keep her knowledge of medical finance up to date will need to be aware of publications which give these facilities. She should ensure these are maintained in the surgery as part of the regular reading of those who find themselves responsible for practice finances.

1   Already referred to, the Red Book, is a valuable source of information and indeed the definitive source of such information. An up-to-date copy should be available in every surgery.
2   The recently published guide, *Making Sense of the New Contract*, from Radcliffe Medical Press interprets the Red Book in a rather more easily-readable manner.
3   Certain medical publications produce relevant articles from time to time: *Medeconomics*, *Pulse*, *Financial Pulse*, *General Practitioner*, and *Doctor Magazine* all operate in this field and should be essential reading for the well-informed practice manager.
4   The doctor in practice wishing to keep up to date on pensions and investments as they affect GPs should obtain the regular bulletins issued by the Medical and Dental Retirement Advisory Service (MADRAS), which are issued free to members. These can be obtained from MADRAS at Hertlands House, Primett Road, Stevenage, Herts SG1 3EE.

5   Some firms of accountants issue up-to-date guides to medical finance
    containing all manner of information concerning accounting and
    taxation topics.
6   *Making Sense of Practice Finance* by John Dean from Radcliffe Medical
    Press is a very useful guide for all those interested in practice finance.

Appendix A: Fees and Allowances for GPs: 1990/91 and 1991/92

		Previous scale to 31 March 1991	1991/92 Scale To 30 November 1991	1991/92 Scale From 1 December 1991
		per annum		
		£	£	£
Practice allowances:				
Maximum for:	Basic (BPA): Full rate	6000	6144	6144
	50% time	3750	3840	3840
	75% time	5125	5247	3840
Designated area:	I	3125	3125	3125
	II	4765	4765	3125
Seniority: Stage	I	400	400	400
Stage	II	2090	2090	2090
Stage	III	4500	4500	4500
Postgraduate Education Allowance (full rate)		2025	2025	2025
Trainee Supervision Grant		4240	4240	4240
Assistant's Allowance:				
	Ordinary	5585	5585	5585
	In designated area	7820	7820	7820
* Associate Allowance (max: 3rd year)		21 250	22 845	23 275
Leave Advance (20% of BPA)		1200	–	–
		Fees per patient		
		£ p		
Capitation fees: Standard:				
Age:	To 64	12.40	13.05	13.30
	65–74	16.30	17.20	17.50
	75 and over	31.45	33.16	33.75
Addition for out-of-hours		2.50		
Deprivation payments:	High level	8.80	9.00	9.05
(per patient)	Medium level	6.65	6.80	6.85
	Low level	5.05	5.65	5.20
New registration		5.80	6.00	6.10
Child health surveillance		5.00	8.35	10.00
Rural practice:	Unit payment	0.224		
Target payments (maximum per doctor):				
Childhood immunizations:	Higher	1800	*	*
	Lower	600	*	*
Pre-school boosters:	Higher	600	*	*
	Lower	200	*	*
Cervical cytology:	Higher	2280	*	*
	Lower	760	*	*

Sessional payments:

Health promotion clinics	45.00	45.00	45.00
Minor surgery (per five operations)	100.00	100.00	100.00
Teaching medical students	10.95	10.95	10.95

Item-of-service fees, etc.:

Night visit fee:	Higher rate	45.00	45.00	45.00
	Lower rate	15.00	15.00	15.00
**Maternity fees				
(obst list: complete service)		150.00	150.00	153.00
Anaesthetic fee		32.20	32.20	32.20
IUCD		42.75	42.75	42.75
Contraception		12.75	12.75	12.75
* Emergency treatment and minor ops		19.05	19.30	19.45
Immediate necessary treatment:				
Up to 15 days		7.30		
More than 15 days		10.95		
Temporary resident:	To 15 days	7.30	7.60	7.80
	Over 15 days	10.95	11.45	11.70
Vaccination:	Lower	3.35	3.35	3.35
	Higher	4.85	4.85	4.85
Dental haemorrhage:	Higher rate	19.20	19.30	19.45
Locum allowance in sickness				
(weekly maximum)		335.00	*	*
Cremation certificates: B&C (each)		25.75	*	*
* Doctors' retainer payment		33.55	*	*

*   Please refer to detailed fees as published from time to time.
** A full scale of maternity fees, depending whether or not the doctor is on the obstetric list, is available from most medical journals.

Appendix B: Current (March 1991) Cost-rent Limits

Building cost limits per practice unit	Rate A (£)	Rate B (£)
One GP	55 100	47 900
Two GPs	100 900	87 700
Three GPs	151 700	132 000
Four GPs	184 300	160 300
Five GPs	217 700	189 300
Six GPs	245 500	213 600
Seven GPs	276 500	240 500
Eight GPs	307 000	266 900
Nine GPs	337 900	293 800
Ten GPs	368 900	320 800
Optional extra rooms:		
offices per m²	502	436
common room per m²	502	436
dispensary per m²	502	436
plus externals	15%	15%
plus professional fees	10–11.5%	10–11.5%
with VAT	17.5%	17.5%
plus planning consent fees	100%	100%
plus approved site cost	100%	100%
Substantial alterations		
combined consulting/examination room	6801	7400

Rate A: For developments (pre-April 1989) and building alterations
Rate B: For new developments from April 1989 (inclusive of VAT)

12   Prescribing

PRESCRIPTION costs and prescribing habits have been a major concern of all governments since the start of the NHS. Many attempts have been made over the years to exert control over the expense of drugs, despite the fact that the UK spends less on pharmaceuticals, whether prescribed by doctors or bought over the counter, than nearly all other developed nations. None of these attempts has had any lasting effect, and few have even had an immediate effect.

Pharmacists have been paid centrally since the inception of the NHS and therefore there is a central record of all pharmaceutical costs at the Prescription Pricing Authority (PPA) in Newcastle upon Tyne. Additionally, the names of all GPs are on their prescription pads so that individual GPs costs can be calculated. Before the PPA was computerized, the only information available for each GP was the total cost of his prescriptions and the number of items prescribed. By dividing the number of items into the total cost, the cost of a Prescribing Unit (PU) could be ascertained for each GP, practice, FHSA, Region and all Regions. The cost for each GP and his practice was compared with those of the FHSA and the Region and these figures were sent to each practice once a year.

The reports were known as PD2s. Any practice that was 25% above the Regional average was visited by the District Medical Officer (DMO) and asked, in consultation with the DMO, to consider how costs could be reduced. These visits had only a limited influence on the reduction of costs and, although they continued, other strategies were tried. The idea of prescribing drugs by the generic name was instituted in the early 1960s and initially caused some concern because of the low standard of production of imported generic drugs. Nevertheless generic prescribing continues to be encouraged, despite initial and considerable protest from the pharmaceutical industry, but the effect on the cost of prescribing, has been limited.

In April 1985, the Department of Health introduced the 'Black List'. A list was published of cough medicines, laxatives and old-fashioned quack remedies which GPs were forbidden to prescribe unless they paid for them personally. This actually did have the desired effect, although it gradually wore off over the following two or three years.

The PPA was finally computerized in 1987, and it then became possible to calculate each GP's costs by category, type of drug and it's use and that information was sent to each GP. Prescribing Analyses and Costs (PACT) was launched and, in August 1988, each GP was sent a filing box in which to store his reports and his first PACT report (covering the costs for

February to April 1988) complete with descriptive notes. Since then reports have been sent every three months, the figures being three months in arrears. The analysis is available at three levels.

Level 1 is a simple quarterly analysis of a practice's prescribing. The data on the first page are an expanded version of the PD2s, listing the prescribing costs, number of items and cost per item numerically and in bar charts. These are practice figures and are compared with data for the local FHSA, the Region and for England.

The next two pages give the practice information on the number of items and their cost under six chapter headings of the BNF; cardiovascular system; musculoskeletal and joint diseases; gastrointestinal system; central nervous system; infections; and respiratory system. These BNF chapters have been chosen because they contain the most costly drugs. All other prescriptions are grouped together as a seventh group.

The fourth page provides information for the individual GP as well as for the practice. This includes the percentage of items that has been prescribed generically, and the number of PUs in the list. As patients over 65 receive, on average, three times as many items as younger patients, allowance is made for this and the number of PUs = (the number of patients under 65) + (3 × the number of patients over 65).

Level 2 draws attention to prescribing costs and shows where they are highest. This Level 2 information is sent automatically to any practice with costs 25% above the local average, or with items under one of the six leading chapter headings which are at least 75% above the local average. However, any practice may request this level of information which is extremely useful for looking at ways of saving, and is not overpowering in the amount of information presented.

Level 3 may be requested by an individual or a practice. If the GP is a trainer, the trainee report comes automatically if some FP10s have been endorsed with a 'D'.

The first three pages of Level 3 repeat those of Level 2. On the fourth and fifth pages the items are divided into 21 therapeutic chapters which correspond with the chapters in the BNF. The total number of items, the total cost, the items and cost per 1000 patients, and the items and cost per 1000 PUs are given for each therapeutic category. Every item that has been dispensed in the quarter is listed on the pages following, with the quantity prescribed and it's cost. The full Level 3 report may run to more than 100 pages! It is useful for audit, but can be overpowering.

The use of PACT data allows the doctor to review his prescribing habits and to make his prescribing more effective, more rational and, all things being equal, more economical. This should be the aim of any responsible GP and is, undoubtedly, the intent of the Department and the Treasury!

When the detail of the 1990 GP Contract was originally made known, the Department indicated that GPs were to be given budgets for their pharmaceutical spending (indicative budgets). GPs were extremely concerned at that time about how they could stay within the constraints of those limits since there are no set limits for patients' demands. Happily, the Department has now thought better of it's original idea and, although it is going to give GPs indicative amounts to aim for, it has dropped the idea of indicative budgets.

Indicative amounts will be set by each FHSA. With the demise of the Regional Medical Service, there is no longer a DMO, and each FHSA has funding to appoint an Independent Medical Adviser (IMA). One of the tasks of the IMA will be to advise on the amount to be set for each GP in consultation with the general manager and the finance manager of the FHSA.

The indicative amounts will be based on the GP's 'historic spend', that is, the amounts spent in previous years, plus an added factor known as the 'uplift' factor. This will be set by the Department to allow for the expected rise in the cost of pharmaceuticals in the coming year. In addition, the GP will be asked to report to the IMA any particularly high cost patients that he may have in order that allowance can be made for the expense. A patient in renal failure, who is having CAPD and being treated with erythropoietin, can add 10% to a normal budget. It is therefore very important to respond to requests from the FHSA for information about high-cost patients.

A GP will be expected to stay within the indicative amount once it has been set for him. If his historic spend has been 25% or more above the FHSA average, he will be visited by the IMA and a lower amount will be negotiated with him making allowance for any high-cost patients. Some FHSAs will visit GPs who are only 10% or 15% above the average.

Although it may seem that there is an intention on the part of the Department to keep greater control over prescribing costs, through the agency of the Regional Health Authority (RHA) and the FHSAs, they nevertheless state that, 'expenditure on drugs prescribed by GPs not in the GP fund-holding scheme will not be cash limited, i.e. there will be no ceiling put on such expenditure'. They also state that, 'The aim of the scheme is not to make arbitrary cuts in the expenditure but to encourage more cost effective prescribing'.

For GP fund-holders a notional indicative prescribing amount will be arrived at in the same way as for non-fund-holders. The notional amount 'will then be adjusted to the true cost of the prescriptions by applying a factor which takes account of the national average discount available to pharmacists and an estimate of the cost containers. The factor will be supplied to RHAs by the Department of Health. Statements of expenditure on drugs sent monthly to RHAs, FHSAs and fund-holders by the PPA will enable monitoring of basic prices, discounts and container costs and the statements will be the basis of charges made on each fund-holder's allocation'. If fund-holders can save on prescribing costs, the money thereby saved can be allocated to buy other services for their patients.

In conclusion it is evident that the practice manager has a considerable role to play in encouraging the GPs to use the information provided so that they may prescribe more effectively and economically.

13   The GP Fund-holding Initiative

The fund-holding pratice

The somewhat radical concept of GPs controlling for the first time large sums of public money and running budgets with all that this implies, was introduced to a somewhat sceptical and unsuspecting world of medical finance in January 1989 with the issue of the White Paper, *Working for Patients*. Since then, a number of amendments have been made to the original proposals, and there was further bulletin issued in December 1989 with a more detailed prospectus which gave additional details, and invited practices to make formal application for fund-holding status.

This legislation has now passed into law in the form of the National Health Service and Community Care Act, 1990.

The first wave of fund-holding proper commenced on 1 April 1991.

Health authorities

The ultimate authorities for administering the scheme are the RHAs of which there are 14 in England and Wales. RHAs are directly responsible to the Department of Health. Separate Authorities operate in Scotland.

FHSAs are likely to have rather closer and more regular contact with practices. They will be responsible, amongst other things, for settlement of costs, payment of invoices and direct supervision of practices.

Qualifying for fund-holding

This is at present voluntary and no practice is being asked to enter the scheme against their will. Applications were originally restricted to partnerships or groups of doctors with 11 000 or more patients, but this has since been reduced to 9000.

Over 800 practices initially registered an interest in entering the scheme, but after the primary process of 'weeding-out', it seemed that some 400 practices would commence as fund-holders. The initial 'first wave' contained some 306 practices nationwide.

It is also clear that a number of practices kept their options open and will decide at a later date whether to enter the 'second wave' on 1 April 1992, or even at a later date. Initial indications are that the 'second wave' fund holders might number about 350 practices.

Selection for the scheme

It is clear already that from the first wave of applicants, a number were rejected as their systems did not fall within accepted guidelines. Although no guarantees can be given, it seems clear that a number of criteria will be taken into account in the selection process, and a practice should be able to organize its management and administration in such a way as will qualify for fund-holding status.

1   The facility already available, or expected to be installed, for information technology, i.e. computerization.
2   The quality of the management of the practice; attitudes of the partners and their general philosophy of commitment to the scheme.
3   Standard of efficiency already in place, including the quality of practice manager, management structure, etc.
4   The number and quality of existing staff and whether they are competent to run a budget.
5   A proper recording system for hospital referrals, including the establishment of existing patterns.
6   Existing records of prescribing.
7   Efficient internal accounting systems and records, including annual accounts.

Formulating the budget

Funds will not, as originally envisaged, by paid direct to the GP or his practice, but will be retained by the FHSA, who will meet bills up to the level of the budget submitted by the practice, or indeed in excess of that figure in exceptional cases. These costs will fall under three main headings.

• Dispensing costs.
• Hospital referrals.
• Ancillary staff costs.

Budgets will initially be set by the RHA, and are subject to negotiation by potential fund-holders. Practices should be prepared to formulate detailed budgets under the headings set out above.

Whilst dispensing costs and hospital referrals will not physically pass through the practice's fund-holding bank account, but be paid directly from FHSA funds, ancillary staff costs will continue to be met from a practice's own accounts, being reimbursed periodically from fund accounts held by the practice for this purpose.

The administration charge

All practices accepted for fund-holding status will have access to a sum of money from which they can meet all amounts necessary, up to an annual maximum, for the administration of the budget. In the initial year, 1990/91, this maximum allowance was £16 000, and presumably this will be available in a preliminary year to those practices who enter as 'the second wave' or subsequent applicants.

The allowance has been set at £33 000 for 1991/92, which will, for the 'first-wave' practices, be the first actual fund-holding year. Of that amount, no more than £1000 may be spent on capital expenditure.

It will be essential for applicants to determine how they propose to use this allowance and this is likely to be included in the overall business plan which the practice will have to submit (see page 195).

An outline of the allocation of a specimen annual administration charge for 1991/92 is set out in Fig. 13.1.

	£	£	£
Staffing expenses: salaries of additional staff			
Budget manager	15 000		
NIC (10.4%)	1560		
		16 560	
Secretarial assistance (part-time)	3000		
Assistant operator (part-time)	4000		
NIC, etc (say)	700		
		7700	24 260
Postage and stationery (est)			740
Computer facility			
Maintenance charges		1200	
Balance of leasing premium		2000	
			3200
Recruitment costs			
Agency fees (part cost)			800 [1]
Professional fees			
Assistance with preparation of annual accounts			3000
Training costs			
Computer training			1000 [1]
			33 000

Notes
[1] These costs likely to be non-recurring.
[2] This is provided for illustration and guidance only: in practice each case would be considered on its merits. Figures should not be assumed to apply to any individual practice.

Figure 13.1 Proposals for allocation of management charge (1991/92).[2]

Staffing and management

It will be highly desirable for practices to formulate and agree a detailed management structure before setting-up their fund-holding procedures. If this is not done, duties to be performed by responsible staff will be unclear and problems will almost certainly arise in this connection. Most practices will wish to recruit a specialist fund project manager who will be responsible for the detailed administration of the budget on a day-to-day basis, and will be responsible directly to the partners.

It will be necessary, particularly, to formalize the roles of the fund manager and the practice manager respectively. There is set out in Fig. 13.2, two separate and alternative management structures which could well apply in a fund-holding practice. These two schemes are by no means the only ones which could be prepared and each practice will decide its own management structure on its merits and taking local conditions into account. What is clear, however, is that any practice not making decisions along these lines could well be storing up potential problems.

Organization chart 1

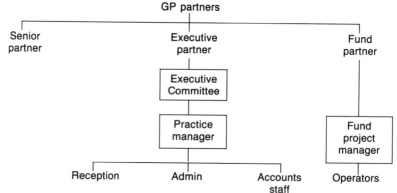

Organization chart 2

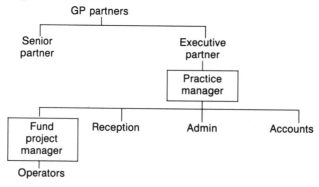

Figure 13.2 Formalization of roles.

Ideally, one partner should be designated by his colleagues to be responsible for the overall supervision of the fund. It is with him that the ultimate responsibility will lie, and he should have a working knowledge of the fund, its accounting, computer and referral systems so that he can take over in times of emergency. Appointed staff can leave at relatively short notice, and it is essential that there is always someone available who is trained and capable of dealing with the day-to-day management of the fund.

Business plans

Practices accepted for the scheme will, as a condition of entry, be required to produce a business plan for several years hence, which will need to be drawn up with professional assistance. These costs can be paid out of the administration charge. The plan will look at the items to be included in the budget and will set these out in some detail. It will look at the future profitability and cash flows of the practice, as well as highlighting strengths and weaknesses. It will also look at such items as the successions in partnership, the role of staff members and the practice manager, outside professional advisers and the like.

The plan, once prepared and agreed, will be an invaluable management tool, and should serve the practice, as a business, in the immediate future and for a number of years.

In some cases, practices may prefer to have such a plan prepared in conjunction with a Business Plan from the Enterprise Initiative Scheme by the Department of Trade and Industry, under which half the cost of such a plan will be paid from Government funds.

Some practices have preferred to draw up the Business Plan themselves, without using outside advice. This may not provide the objective and detached view required, and if done to save money could turn out to be a false economy.

The manual of accounts

The GP fund-holders' manual of accounts was issued by the Department of Health in September 1990. This is an extremely complex document which lists the accounting requirements for the fund-holding facility, and sets out in several appendices the actual bookkeeping entries required.

Whilst it is true that a great deal of these entries will be dealt with by the computer program, it will be necessary for fund managers and operators to understand how the system works, and they will need to have a working knowledge of theoretical double-entry bookkeeping, which is the overall system in use.

With regard to the organization and staffing of the fund-holding facility, the practice will need to ensure that there are clear guidelines for those who will be responsible for:

- the regular input of data;
- the checking and approval of accounts for payment;
- implementing the necessary control procedures;
- control of the fund-holding bank account;
- preparation of monthly and annual accounts.

This chapter does not fully detail all the complex requirements of the *Manual of accounts*. Fund managers are advised to study this publication carefully and to take advantage of the numerous training opportunities which are available. These are offered not only by RHAs, but by computer software houses and other commercial sources. These training costs will be payable out of the annual administration charge.

The Department of Health (DoH) helpline

In order to assist practices and managers in understanding the *Manual of accounts* and to provide immediate explanation, the Department of Health has established a helpline which can be used during normal working hours: telephone: 0483 573853, fax: 0483 578880. The helpline is restricted to interpretation and explanation of the *Manual of accounts* and is not available for more general enquiries on the fund-holding facility.

Hospital referrals

One of the most complex parts of the control of the budget will be that concerning patient referrals to hospitals.

It is essential that all data introduced to the system is correct as this will have to be checked against hospital invoices, and approved for payment by the practice.

There should be in force a system of passwords to ensure that only authorized entries and referrals can be made.

Detailed advice should be taken on this aspect of the budget.

Annual accounts

Regardless of the date to which the practice prepares its own financial accounts, the annual accounts of the fund-holding facility must be drawn up to 31 March each year. These must be submitted to the FHSA within six weeks of that date. This is a deadline which may be extremely difficult to meet, particularly in view of the anticipated delays in obtaining invoices from provider units such as local hospitals.

At this level the accounts themselves are not required to have an annual audit, but it seems clear that there will be an independent check on these every three years by the Audit Commission, who will also have access to the financial books of the practice if required.

The FHSAs will prepare summaries of the accounts of each fund-holder within their area, and at this level the accounts will be audited on an annual basis.

Computer systems

In early 1991 a number of computer software programs were introduced. At the time of writing these are being perfected and staff are being trained in their use. Fund managers are strongly advised to seek the training opportunities offered by the software companies.

Generous grants are available for fund-holding practices for the acquisition of their computer systems. See Fig. 13.3 for the scales of computer reimbursements.

The announcement of an enhanced rate of reimbursement for fund-holding practices will ease their concern over the likely cost of purchasing the hardware and the special computer programs which will be necessary.

Such a practice with 20 000 or more patients will attract the reimbursement of purchase costs up to £15 375, with a further scale applying to running costs and maintenance.

Maximum payments according to the list size of a partnership or group practice (includes element of reimbursement available to all GPs).

List size	Systems purchase upgrading[1]	Systems leasehold/ upgrading[2]	Maintenance[3]
9000–10 000	£10 425	£2605	£1565
10 001–12 000	£12 375	£3095	£1855
12 001–14 000	£13 125	£3280	£1970
14 001–16 000	£13 875	£3470	£2080
16 001–18 000	£14 625	£3655	£2195
18 001–20 000	£15 375	£3845	£2305

NB All payments include VAT

[1] The maximum amount payable for computer systems purchased and upgrades purchased for the duration of the scheme.
[2] The maximum annual payment for the duration of the scheme.
[3] The maximum annual payment for the duration of the scheme.

Figure 13.3 Computer costs.

Under and overspending

Where a practice overspends its budget, this will be allowed to continue for a year, although in the event of serious overspending for a more lengthy period, the practice may be withdrawn from the scheme.

If the budget is underspent (i.e. in surplus) at the end of the year, the practice can retain this to cover expenses on developing the practice. This will count towards such expenditure as medical and surgical equipment, surgery improvements and repairs, and numerous other items.

Practices should not embark upon expenditure of this nature unless they have established that a surplus has indeed been generated, and that this has been accepted by the RHA.

Such surpluses, if unspent, can be carried forward for a maximum of four years. Fund-holding is an initiative which gives practices an opportunity for ensuring improved treatment facilities for their practice. It is not designed to generate additional income for the GP or his practice. From the practice's point of view it will be a complex and difficult system to administer, and it is essential that before embarking on the scheme the practice is aware of all the obligations involved, and the exact manner in which the project will be managed, financed and administered.

It will require an organized and business-like approach. Only those who are adequately equipped and committed – both mentally and physically – to embark on such a project should even contemplate doing so.

14   Managing Patients

Introduction

IN this final chapter the implications of management are explored in relation to patients. It is important that practice managers see their role as central to patient care and not merely in a limited and restricted way.

It should be clear by now that primary health teams are complex organizations—indeed it has been said that if someone had wanted to devise a more complicated grouping of people they could hardly have done better. There is usually more than one director, or partner, and some of them may not agree with the others. Some of the team members, including the practice manager, are employed by the partners, whilst others are employed by the health authority or health board. It is important therefore that practice managers understand how to make teams work as effectively as possible.

One of the ways to facilitate this is by the use of objectives already referred to in an earlier chapter. Hardly any practices have objectives that are written down; many doctors and nurses, when asked what they are trying to do, have the greatest difficulty in answering the question. They seem to go to work for many years and never really think through what they are trying to achieve or whether they are being effective.

Writing down the practice objectives has several advantages. First, it will make the team members think through what they are aiming for. Second, the process itself, if properly conducted, brings the various team members together. Third, it enables the practice manager to manage, once she knows what the targets are. Finally, it means that the work of the practice can be audited or measured.

At Sonning Common Health Centre all the staff were involved in compiling the practice aims and objectives a few years ago. Some areas were precise and easy whilst others were more nebulous. Every so often they have to be reviewed: some may be out of date and others can be sharpened up. The 1990 GP Contract contains certain objectives that have to be adhered to and these need careful study by all concerned.

Promoting the practice

In the past, practices did little to promote themselves or to tell patients about the services on offer. This was partly because there has been little competition for patients in the NHS in the past 30 years and partly because advertising is not allowed under General Medical Council rules.

Things are now changing. It has been accepted for some time that as patients have become better informed, they are entitled to know how a practice operates and what it can provide. Many mothers want to know for example whether there are antenatal and child health clinics, elderly people are anxious to know how to get a home visit and everyone needs to know what to do in an emergency. So in the past few years an increasing number of practices have produced practice leaflets or brochures which are available to patients who are registered or who are thinking of registering with the practice.

Competition

One of the main themes of the Government's 1989 proposals for the Health Service was that competition should be a feature of NHS care and that this would apply to general medical as well as specialist practice. Since April 1990 the percentage of a GP's income related to the number of patients on the list has risen and changing doctors has been made much easier: if patients wish to change they merely have to take their medical cards to another doctor without seeking permission from their previous doctor, even if they are not moving house.

This means that practices in some parts of the country may start to compete for patients and even those practices that do not wish to increase their list size will want to ensure that patients are not lured away. A good practice manager will pay careful attention to all aspects of the practice that affect its image and everyone will need to be on his or her toes to make sure that the service is first class. Table 14.1 contains a check list of things to consider.

Table 14.1 Check list for practice image.

Reception area and layout
Notice boards and posters
Practice leaflets
Receptionists' manner and dress
Arrangements for appointments
Repeat prescription system
Waiting room
Out-of-hours telephones
Car parking

Practice image

Under the terms of the 1990 GP Contract doctors have to make sure that the reception area is not only adequate but that patients can talk to receptionists in reasonable privacy. Make sure that notice boards look reasonably attractive, that they are not full of outdated information and that the contents are helpful rather than punitive and dictatorial.

Practice leaflets should be readily available and attractively designed. From April 1990 certain information is compulsory[1] and is shown in Table 14.2.

Table 14.2 Mandatory information for practice leaflets.

Names, qualifications and year of birth or first qualification of doctor(s)
Sex of doctor(s)
Surgery times
Information on how to make appointments
Home visit arrangements
Emergency call arrangements
Off duty arrangements
Repeat prescription (and dispensing) arrangements
Clinic times
Details of staff employed
Other services
Patient participation activities
Geographical area covered
Access for disabled

Source: *Health Departments of Great Britain: The 1990 Contract*

The receptionist is the first member of the staff the patient normally sees. As well as being welcoming it is important that receptionists look nice. A number of practices are now moving away from uniforms and white coats to standardized blouses and skirts. At Sonning Common Health Centre there is a different colour for each day of the week so that although each member of staff can wear the clothes that suit her best there is some co-ordination. It is helpful if staff wear name badges and some practices now have photographs of all their staff in the waiting room showing their name and what they do.

The waiting room should be friendly with up-to-date magazines and flowers. Some doctors are dispensing with loudspeakers, lights and buzzers and are calling in patients personally. Not only does this make the initial contact more personal but it reduces the conveyor belt image.

Informed receptionists

Many receptionists come to recognize the regular patients and know many of their names. Anything that helps the staff to take a personal interest is important. Whilst it is not appropriate for receptionists to know the details of someone's medical problems, asking after relatives in hospital or recognizing someone who is newly widowed will be appreciated. A few practices have boards in the office showing which patients are in hospital and listing all recent deaths. Receptionists need to be able to recognize symptoms that may indicate serious illness and therefore need urgent attention from the doctor.

Interview with new patients

A few practices offer routine consultations for all patients who are registering with the practice and since April 1990 this attracted an additional fee. The purpose of such interviews is to allow the doctor or nurse to start to get to know the patient and to carry out a simple prevention check. But the receptionist too should be able to offer a short interview to explain how the practice works rather than merely handing over a leaflet. A few minutes with a new patient, quietly and confidentially, is time well spent and pays dividends in building a sound relationship. Such sessions will set the tone for the practice.

Advertising

Whilst providing factual information about services is considered important, advertising goes against the traditions of the medical profession. Although the Government would like to see advertising to promote competition the General Medical Council is not in favour of such a development.

In its advice to the profession[2] the GMC states 'Patients are entitled to protection from misleading promotional advertising'. 'Canvassing by a doctor for the purpose of obtaining patients . . . is unethical' and 'it is improper for a doctor to disparage . . . the professional skill . . . of any other doctor'. The Council does accept, however, that factual information should be readily available. The important point is that all information whether by mouth or in writing should be accurate and should not imply that the practice is superior in skill to the one down the road. The distinction between what constitutes information as opposed to advertising may become rather more blurred in the future.

Accessibility and availability

Whatever the role, receptionist, nurse, health visitor or doctor, members of the primary health care team are united in having one major aim: the delivery of a quality service that is accessible to all who need it. 'Of course we are accessible', some might state hastily. 'Open from 8.30 a.m, until 6.00 p.m. Monday to Friday, Saturday morning as well; a reception desk and three telephone lines manned all of that time; appointment sessions spread throughout the day; an answering machine for out-of-hours emergency calls; 24 hours a day, 365 days of the year—that's us, pretty wonderful!' In fact such statements tell little about a practice. Indeed many practices are centres of excellence and clearly accessible but for reasons far and beyond 'appointments' and 'telephones', etc. Fortunately, studies undertaken have shown that on the whole access is satisfactory. In this context 'satisfactory' seems to hint at mediocrity; not bad, but could be better. What are the factors then, that have to be taken into account to ensure that patients receive the type of service that is more than merely satisfactory?

External factors

Many factors govern access, some of which are completely outside the control of the practice. None the less, an understanding and awareness of barriers, both real and potential, is essential. To enable the practice manager to assist with planning and making decisions she will require grass-roots knowledge of what it is really like for patients to access the service. Table 14.3 gives some examples.

Table 14.3 Factors affecting accessibility.

1	Public transport system
2	Car ownership
3	Possession of a telephone
4	Availability of public telephones (and are they in working order?)
5	Distances to and from the surgery
6	Elderly and infirm patients
7	Young parents with small children—in particular single parents
8	Patients who experience difficulties in getting time off work
9	Patients who have little or no knowledge of practice arrangements
10	Cultural and language barriers

The list in Table 14.3 is not definitive but these types of issues allow the practice valuable insight into the type of hurdles that can make life very difficult for the patient. It is little wonder that patients who are ill or anxious sometimes demonstrate aggressive behaviour, or simply give up any struggle at the first hurdle, complain to all but not to the practice, or simply suffer in silence until crisis point.

There is little the practice manager can do to influence such factors, other than highlight a problem area, but it does also demonstrate again the many difficulties faced by the receptionists and the support required.

Internal factors

Let us now take a look at some other factors influencing accessibility, this time once the patient has arrived at the surgery premises, or has dialled the practice telephone number. 'Piece of cake from now on'—or is it? Here are some further examples, but all of them clearly under the control of the practice.

1   The premises:
    Steps, ramps, doors and whether they open easily or are heavily weighted, corridors, toilets that are accessible to patients in wheelchairs, areas for prams, pushchairs and bicycles, clear signs.

2   Telephones:
    There is little point in having four telephone lines and four instruments if there is no arrangement for 'hands' to answer the calls (i.e. staffing levels). Two receptionists can only answer two telephone lines at any one time.

3   Appointments:
    The number of consulting hours per day to be in relation to list size. A partner absent on holiday and another attending a course may reduce the number of available appointments to a level that is far below that which would be considered acceptable and reasonable.

4   Workload:
    Systems for monitoring the peaks and troughs of the practice workload—not only the 'flu' epidemic in the middle of winter—but systems that will enable careful monitoring of day-to-day and daily work. Simple 'counts' and graphs will suffice to enable the practice manager and other members of the practice to make plans and take decisions based on fact. A busy time for telephone calls may be 8.30 a.m. until 10.30 a.m. in one practice, whilst in another quite a different time of the day, such information being significant in determining staff cover.

5 Urgent requests:
   Procedures should be discussed, agreed, set down, and understood by
   all. A distressed patient, or relative, will be comforted by the fact his or
   her request is being dealt with in a calm, efficient and orderly manner,
   ensuring that the patient receives the help that is required, as quickly
   as possible. Telephone systems that play music to the patient who is
   'holding on', and frantically trying to speak to the doctor are felt by
   many to be inappropriate.

6 Home visits:
   Guidelines, once again communicated and understood by all will
   undoubtedly be helpful.

7 Telephone interruptions:
   Are patients able to ask to speak to their doctor at any point during the
   day—is this fair to the patient who has made an appointment and has
   the consultation interrupted, once, or perhaps twice in the space of a
   few minutes? Can a busy hospital colleague be asked to 'telephone
   back'? Is this reasonable?

Again, these are only examples and are by no means definitive but merely
set out some areas of the service that are clearly under the control of the
practice.

All of this still leaves an important question to be asked. If the practice
manager is sensitive and aware of the community her practice serves, and
has organized and managed the systems and services within the practice to
be truly accessible, how can she ensure all the arrangements are conveyed
to the patients? Quite simply, she cannot but there are many positive steps
that can be taken, or opportunities to act upon. Interviews with new
patients have already been mentioned as particularly important occasions
and such patients must be made particularly welcome.

Practice boundaries

GPs may work as single-handed practitioners or in groups of ten or more
with practice premises and offices that range in simplicity or sophistication
from a single receptionist making appointments to a complex team of
secretaries and receptionists supported by the most modern information
technology system.

Such is the diversity of general practice and so too are the areas and
boundaries in which doctors will look after patients. A single-handed
practitioner on a remote Hebridean island, or rural Yorkshire Dale may
look after a few hundred patients. In these circumstances two home
visits may be a long distance apart with possibly an hour or two spent

travelling from one to the other—a particular problem when considering 'accessibility'. On the other hand, a partnership of seven doctors may be responsible for 12 000 patients in an area of only one square mile. Consider the density of housing schemes and multi-rise blocks.

GPs are 'independent contractors' and when signing the contract with the FHSA (Health Board in Scotland) will be requested to define the area in which the practitioner agrees to be responsible for patients. Doctors may choose, and indeed some do, to accept patients from a very broad area, i.e. north of a city, south of a city, encompassing many miles, whilst others may be strict and adhere rigidly to very clear boundaries. Whatever areas are chosen, these must be defined to the FHSA (Health Board).

A good idea is to highlight the area on a map and have this placed in a strategic position. Mrs Brown may plead with 'her' doctor to remain on the list though moving out of the defined area. This is a difficult decision no doubt for the doctor who has looked after Mrs Brown and her family for many years, and is compounded by the fact that Mrs Brown adds 'promise not to call you out—ever!' This is problematical and emotional for both, but the fact remains that the service is organized and maintained for the benefit of *all* patients. A doctor on duty who has to travel through the centre of the city to an outlying area is not very accessible to the patient well within the defined area who may be having a heart attack.

Both the lack of practice boundary definition, or defining it and not communicating this to receptionists or other professional colleagues will cause endless confusion. The practice manager needs to be absolutely clear on the policy and may need to set up a special meeting to convey to all members of the team:

- the geographical area of the practice;
- whether or not the practice will make exceptions, and what these are;
- whether particular doctors' lists are closed or open;
- procedure for accepting patients from other practices.

General practice *is* diverse—indeed it is that diversity that makes it so exciting—but it does mean that there should not be hard and fast rules, only guidelines. Practices, people and communities are different. Each practice must be encouraged to establish policy, and once established to record it. It is all very well to state 'we do it this way in our practice' but to be fully effective it has to be written down. At the beginning of this chapter we emphasized the need for objectives and Table 14.4 gives some sample objectives on accessibility.

Table 14.4 Sample objectives for accessibility.

1 All patients should be able to see the doctor of their choice within three days.

2 All patients requesting appointments for the same day should be able to see one of the doctors on that day.

3 No patient should have to wait more than 20 minutes to be seen after their appointment time.

4 All patients should be able to speak on the telephone to doctors, nurses and health visitors without having to ring back more than once.

5 All patients should be able to speak to the duty doctor on the telephone out of hours without having to make more than two calls.

Drugs and prescriptions

Each year doctors write or sign thousands of prescriptions and the cost constitutes a significant percentage of the cost of the NHS as a whole. The Government White Paper proposals for general practice include some designed to 'place downward pressure on expenditure on drugs' and will involve budgeting[3]. Practice managers also need to understand the legal aspects of prescribing.

Drug information

In the past, GPs have been free to prescribe generally whatever they have felt is appropriate for their patients regardless of cost. The main guide is the British National Formulary which is published regularly by the British Medical Association and the Royal Pharmaceutical Society and is issued free to all doctors. It lists all the drugs in general use by the basic (generic name) and also lists for each individual drug the various proprietary brands and manufacturers. For example, under amoxycillin (a common antibiotic) there is amoxycillin (non-proprietary), Almodan (Berk), Amoxil (Bencard) and Augmentin (Beecham). In general generic drugs are cheaper than proprietary versions and doctors are encouraged to prescribe the former.

The other common reference manual is MIMS (Monthly Index of Medical Specialties) sent free to all GPs and containing all the proprietary drugs. Both publications also show costs. For example, the BNF shows basic net prices: the actual cost to the NHS is greater because of overhead allowances and professional fees to retail pharmacists and dispensing doctors.

Drug categories

Some drugs can be bought over the counter (OTC) as well as being prescribable by doctors and many are cheaper when bought directly, if the patient would otherwise pay a prescription charge. One example is chlorpheniramine (or Piriton, which is the better known proprietary name) for hay fever. Other drugs can only be authorized by a doctor and can only be obtained with a prescription. For example, in the UK all antibiotics come into this category.

Because of the dangers of addiction certain drugs are Controlled Drugs and subject to special rules. For these drugs the doctor must write the whole prescription himself (computer-printed prescriptions or those written by other people will not do) and this has to include the total quantity of the drug in words and figures. Obviously morphine and heroin come into this group but so also do other pain killers like Diconal and Equagesic. Some of these drugs are subject to special requirements for storage and registers so that they can all be accounted for.

A few years ago, in order to reduce costs, the Government introduced a black list of drugs which are no longer prescribable on the NHS. None of these drugs are essential but if a patient wishes to have them they have to be issued on a private prescription.

Safeguards

Many drugs are powerful agents and many have potentially serious side effects. Patients should not allow medicines prescribed for them to be taken by others. Equally, practices should make sure that prescriptions waiting for collection are under the control of receptionists and cannot be collected from racks in the entrance lobby. Prescription pads need to be kept under lock and key when not in use and should never be left lying around, nor should blank forms be pre-signed.

Dispensing doctors

The vast majority of patients take their prescriptions to a retail pharmacist for dispensing. But around 10% of GPs are dispensing doctors. This is to provide a service to patients in rural areas where pharmacies are not readily available. In these practices when patients register with the doctor they may also register for dispensing: normally these patients must live more than a mile from the nearest pharmacy as the crow flies. In these practices special security arrangements will need to be made. The dispensing practice operates in a similar way to a retail pharmacy: the drugs are purchased from wholesale suppliers and each month the prescriptions issued have to be sent in for payment.

Prescribing information

Every quarter, each GP is sent a summary of his or her prescribing costs which show, for each main group of drugs, how the doctors' and practice's costs compare with the FHSA or Health Board and the national average. Under the PACT system doctors can also request more detailed analyses. Level 2 shows the main costs in each drug group and level 3 itemizes all prescriptions. There is an enormous range of costs between the cheapest and most expensive prescribers which is not entirely explained. Whilst in general most costs could be reduced with no disadvantages to patients there are exceptions.

Drug representatives

Drug information of a different kind comes from representatives of pharmaceutical companies and these representatives seek appointments with doctors. Their objective is to provide doctors with information about their company's products. Representatives' material varies from the frankly promotional to reasonably balanced presentations and many representatives now have non-promotional video films. There are also fringe benefits for practices in the form of such things as Biros and note pads.

An increasing number of GPs are not prepared to see representatives because they prefer to obtain all their drug information from the unbiased sources. It is important for practice managers to establish with the partners exactly what their policies are.

Prescribing budgets

Under the Government's proposals for the NHS already referred to[3], each practice is being given an indicative budget. This will be based largely on the previous years' levels although for higher than average practices some reductions will be made. In the words of the working paper report 'the practice will need an estimated monthly profile of expenditure and will need to devise . . . local policies for effective and economic prescribing within budget. The practice will need a monitoring system to compare its prescribing costs with the budget profile'. FHSAs will have to receive aggregated returns.

Whilst the money in the budget is merely indicative and will not be processed through the practice, the partners will have to explain the reason for any divergence from the budget. So it will be important that an effective up-to-date monitoring system is working.

Repeat prescriptions

This is the area of prescribing that impinges the most on practice administration at the moment. It is important that the system operates efficiently and effectively. Many repeat prescriptions are handwritten by secretaries and receptionists which in theory can produce problems because administrative staff cannot know the implications of what they are writing. Some practices do not have an automatic check system that prevents patients collecting prescriptions without ever seeing a doctor.

Drury has reviewed repeat prescribing[4] and his criteria for an effective system are shown in Table 14.5.

Table 14.5   Repeat prescribing system objectives.

1   Prescriptions should be obtainable within 24 hours of ordering.

2   Preparation should be written with meticulous accuracy without errors.

3   There should be a built-in recall system.

4   The medical records should show what drugs are being taken and when the last supply was obtained.

5   The system should be as simple and cheap as possible.

6   The system should enable the doctors to audit their prescribing.

7   It should be possible to check compliance.

There are three manual methods for issuing repeat prescriptions in common use as described by Drury. First, the patient may hold a repeat prescription card which is used both as the record and the ordering system. Second, the practice may use a special repeat prescription register. Third, a regular prescription record may be in the patient's main record and this can be combined with one of the other two methods. This last method comes closest to meeting Drury's criteria.

Nowadays, however, most modern practices are using microcomputers to run their repeat prescribing. They are rapid, legible and accurate and automatically update the medical record when drugs are issued. Recall dates can easily be entered and audits carried out. The computer prints a patient-held record which is renewed each time prescriptions are processed. Pritchard, Low and Whalen have provided a useful small review of repeat prescribing[5].

Computer-issued prescriptions

Some doctors now issue all their prescriptions by computers and printers in their consulting rooms. The BNF lists the points that should be borne in mind and the FHSA or Health Board will need to be satisfied that the system meets certain criteria.

Managing the practice population

One of the most important features of the UK system of primary health care is the patient registration system. Because all patients have to register with an individual doctor, and because re-registering causes the patient to be removed from the previous doctor's list, practices can identify at any one time for whom they have responsibility. In most other parts of the world this facility does not exist and many overseas doctors and their staff look with envy at our system.

In the early years of the NHS many practices were slow to recognize the benefits of this arrangement. Gradually the more progressive ones realized that they needed this information in order to provide a more sophisticated system of care and, equally important, to be able to start to measure how effectively some of that care was being provided. With the introduction of the 1990 GP Contract[1] practices will have to have detailed statistics based on their practice lists if they are to claim some of their income.

There are various reasons why this information is needed, apart from purely financial ones. First, it enables practices to identify groups of patients for whom certain procedures are appropriate or necessary. Second, it enables practices to work out what the demand for its services is likely to be and whether that demand may change. Third, it shows the practice how well it is doing in providing services by calculating percentages of patients who have received the services. We shall return to these themes in more detail subsequently.

The age–sex register

At the heart of the system is the age–sex register. Basically, this is a mechanism by which all the patients can be grouped according to their age and sex.

There are various ways in which the register can be established. Many are held on card indexes: each patient has a card on which is entered their name, address, date of birth and sometimes other information such as their NHS number. The cards are in two colours, one for each sex, and are filed by year of birth. So, for example, if you wish to find all the boys aged ten and under it is possible to lift out the appropriate batches of cards. It is also possible to put coloured tags on the top of the cards to identify patients with particular characteristics, such as those that are housebound or who have a particular disease.

An alternative system to the card index is a loose leaf folder where all patients are listed page by page according to their sex and year of birth.

Whilst these systems will work they are time-consuming and cumbersome. There is much work involved in writing cards for each new patient and then copying the information off again when a particular group is being circulated or assessed. Practices with high turnovers are constantly writing new cards and tearing up old ones. Moreover, because extracting information is such a laborious process, most practices never get round to counting batches of cards and establishing what proportion of patients have been immunized, had smears taken and so on. Some practices have been maintaining manual age–sex registers as a kind of ritual but, when questioned, the staff are unable to say exactly what they are being used for. There is no question that with the advent of powerful microcomputers the only sensible way to handle data relating to thousands of patients is on a computer and all practices should now be contemplating this. It means that one registration entry automatically incorporates the name in the register but much more importantly, it enables rapid searches to be carried out, not only identifying groups of patients, but linking it to a large amount of other data.

Whilst simple systems will be able to hold the basic register there is much to be said for installing one of the more sophisticated GP systems which enables cross-linking of information.

Creating the register

In the past, doctors and staff waded laboriously along the shelves copying the information from each patient record, and there is much to be said for starting in this way because it enables the practice to check the accuracy of their list as they go. Some practices have then compared their results with the FHSA or Health Board registers and discovered they had patients for whom they were not being paid.

Nowadays, many FHSAs are able to provide the age–sex register from their own central computer system, and this is clearly an advantage in saving time although it may still be advantageous to do some cross-checking.

A detailed information folder on age–sex registers is available from the Central Sales Office at the Royal College of General Practitioners.

The disease index

This is an index which identifies patients who have a particular disease or problem and once again can be held on a card index or in a folder. Diseases which are most commonly entered are long-term ones such as diabetes, rheumatoid arthritis and epilepsy, or important past problems such as coronary thrombosis. This enables particular groups of patients to be looked at to see how well their care is being provided. Practices with the more sophisticated computer systems have the facility built in for every medical problem and a whole list can be searched for any medical condition in a matter of seconds.

Unless a computer system which holds every patient's medical summary is being installed, each index has to be created by doctors remembering to enter patients as they see them or, for those conditions involving continuous medication, from repeat prescription requests. The experience of those of us who visit large numbers of practices is that doctors are generally poor at remembering to keep disease indices up-to-date. Practice managers would be well advised to find ways of bypassing doctors by training staff to identify patients with new significant problems from hospital letters, discharge summaries and clinical records. This applies as much to keeping medical summaries up-to-date as it does to the disease index.

In the next section we look at the uses of the age–sex register and the disease index.

Health promotion and preventive medicine

Over the past two decades a major and important shift has taken place in the service provided by GPs and their colleagues in the primary health team. The shift is from a purely responsive service where patients come with their problems to one where the doctors and nurses initiate activities that are designed to prevent problems in the future. The reasons for this change stem partly from the alterations made to GPs' fees and allowances in the mid-sixties, and partly from increased knowledge about risk factors for disease, especially heart attacks and stroke. Practice managers and their staff should be intimately involved in these developments and further involvement has followed with the 1990 GP Contract.

Prevention activities

Primary care prevention activities can be broadly divided into two sorts. The first is health education which is largely to do with advice about life-style in such areas as eating, smoking and alcohol. The second is procedural and involves activities that doctors and nurses carry out such as immunization or taking cervical smears.

Health education

As far as health education goes, obviously doctors and nurses (especially health visitors) spend much of their ordinary consulting time in giving patients advice. But there are now some key issues that should be raised with all adults because of their health significance and these are shown in Table 14.6.

Table 14.6 Key areas for health education.

Diet
Smoking
Alcohol intake
Exercise
Accident prevention

Smoking causes something like 100 000 premature deaths a year in Britain and it has been calculated that there are perhaps 28 000 extra deaths a year from excess alcohol consumption[6]. Smoking and high cholesterol levels (linked with high levels of saturated fat intake) are two major risk factors for heart attacks and stroke—two of the biggest killers.

Health education and advice is provided in a number of different ways. Many doctors spend time in consultations covering these issues whilst Well-Man and Well-Woman and family planning clinics are obvious places. It is also important, however, to have a ready and comprehensive supply of leaflets covering different subjects and waiting room posters which should be attractive and limited in number. At Sonning Common Health Centre there is now a patients' library under the supervision of one of the receptionists and some practices now use video films in the waiting area.

Procedures

The most important procedures are shown in Table 14.7.

Table 14.7 Key preventive procedures.

Child development checks
Immunization
Cervical cytology
Blood pressure measurement
German measles immunity

Virtually all of these can be carried out by suitably trained nurses. Immunization includes routine injections for children (diphtheria, tetanus, whooping cough, polio, mumps, German measles and measles), tetanus boosters for adults, influenza vaccination for those at risk and other vaccines for foreign travel. In general the immunizations are effective and the serious side effects few. However, UK rates for measles and whooping cough have been poor in the past and the previous policy of giving German measles (rubella) vaccine to teenage girls has not worked very well either.

Raised blood pressure, especially when associated with smoking and high cholesterol levels, is an important risk factor for heart attack and stroke and needs lowering with drugs in some patients. Cervical smears can detect pre-cancerous cells in the neck of the womb (cervix) and one of the main reasons why women still die from cervical cancer is because many of these women have never had a smear.

Targets

Earlier in this book the importance of objectives in management was stressed and at the beginning of this chapter the need for objectives for patient care was underlined again. Preventive medicine is one of the easier parts of clinical care in which to define objectives because generally it is clear what needs to be done. Some of these objectives are now part of the 1990 GP Contract. For example, in order to attract maximum payments for child immunization a 90% immunization rate is needed and for cervical cytology an 80% rate is needed for women aged 25–64. Practices should therefore decide if this is what they are aiming for. Regular health promotion checks every three years will be part of the doctor's contract and these will include a blood pressure check and an enquiry about smoking and alcohol.

Regardless of what the contract requires practices should nevertheless set out their objectives for prevention which in some cases will include specific targets.

Opportunistic screening

There are two ways of ensuring that preventive activities get done, whether in health education or procedural. One is to take the opportunity when the patient comes in for something else—the opportunistic method. The other is to send for patients—screening.

Both methods are needed in practice since neither method will be adequate on its own. Although most patients will be seen during two to three years, some will not and in any case it is not always possible to deal with preventive activities in every consultation. Equally, sending for patients does not produce a 100% response. But a combination of the two seems to be the answer—'opportunistic screening' is the phrase coined by Lawrence[7].

It is important to make sure that the language of letters sent to patients is understandable and friendly: doctors are usually not the best people to draft them. A computer will not only identify the patients but produce a personalized letter. Practices with significant numbers of patients from ethnic minorities or with public transport problems may have to adapt their arrangements to make them effective.

Teamwork

Nowhere is good teamwork more important than in prevention. Since much can be done by nurses and health visitors and the administrative staff they are the key people in sending for patients and checking whether targets are being reached.

Many practices have used the services of a nurse facilitator, a method pioneered in Oxford some years ago[8]. Facilitators, who are now employed by many health authorities, are available to advise practices on how to set up health checks carried out by the practice nurses, mainly in relation to risk factors for heart disease and stroke.

Records

The age – sex register has already been described. Many computerized practices now have a regular schedule so that, for example, patients due for cervical smears are sent for each month, pre-school booster children every quarter, and those due for tetanus boosters every other month.

It is also important that the individual patient records clearly show what has been done and what is needed. A special prevention sheet is usually the answer so that the doctor or nurse can see at a glance the current state of play. If the information on alcohol, smoking, or blood pressure is buried in stacks of paper, no-one is going to start looking for it when there are more patients to be seen.

The practice manager should ensure that regular statistics are produced so that all team members can see how well they are doing: this is where computerization is really the only option. The VAMP system now has a prevention search programme which automatically produces a whole range of data including blood pressure and smoking statistics at the touch of a button.

Chronic disease and long-term problems

The management of chronic disease and long-term problems is fast following prevention and health promotion as one of the main developing areas of primary health care. There is plenty of evidence to show that these problems are not supervised as well as they might be because of organizational deficiencies, and that the long-term complications of diseases such as diabetes may be reduced by careful attention to control.

Whilst the medical management of such disorders is a matter for doctors and nurses the practice manager will have an increasing role in planning and auditing care and providing feedback to the doctors and nurses on their performance. The common diseases that are likely to be suitable for such developments are shown in Table 14.8.

Table 14.8 Some common chronic diseases.

Angina pectoris

Asthma

Diabetes mellitus

Eczema

Epilepsy

Hypertension

Osteoarthritis

Rheumatoid arthritis

Thyroid disorders

Protocols

If the practice manager is to be able to help the doctors and nurses audit their care she will need access to protocols that set out what is being attempted. In the same way that managers need objectives and targets, so doctors and nurses need clinical objectives or protocols that lay down agreed ways of proceeding. Unfortunately, many practices do not have such protocols and the practice manager may have an important role in stimulating such a development.

Protocols vary in detail from mere outlines to sophisticated lists. They need to be created by the doctors and should reflect published medical evidence and also patients' views and needs. For example, if a patient on treatment for high blood pressure gets objectionable side effects from the drugs those side effects may be more of a problem than the risks of leaving the blood pressure alone: the protocol should reflect this. Protocols need to be pragmatic and reflect the real world rather than some ideal but unattainable situation. Here are three examples:

'Before starting a patient on treatment for hypertension, the blood pressure must have been taken at least three times'.

'Each patient newly diagnosed with epilepsy will normally be counselled in the following ten areas'.

'Each patient with suspected asthma will normally measure a series of peak flow readings three times a day for ten days'.

A detailed look at protocol construction has been described by Hasler, Schofield and Barnes[9].

Records

The disease index has already been mentioned. Of equal importance are special record sheets in the patient's individual clinical file. This enables information to be transferred between different doctors and nurses and enables the progress of the patient to be seen easily. It also reminds doctors and nurses what is in the protocol. Most chronic disease record sheets are in the form of flow sheets and the ones in use at Sonning Common Health Centre for epilepsy and blood pressure are shown in Figs 14.1 and 14.2. The epilepsy record reminds the doctors of the important areas to be discussed with the patient whilst the blood pressure record reminds the doctor of the steps to be taken in assessing whether to start treatment. These same flow sheets can also be used by the practice manager and her staff to check whether the appropriate steps have been followed.

For example, it is possible from the disease index to identify all patients newly diagnosed with a certain disease in the previous year and then to see what proportion have records containing flow sheets and which entries have (or have not) been made.

For those diseases where regular examinations and tests have numerical values such as blood pressure or blood sugar levels it is possible to use the computer to carry out more rapid and comprehensive analyses.

Clinics

Traditionally, most general practice care has been given in individual consultations. But there is now an increasing number of practices who provide care for some conditions in a specially organized clinic session. Antenatal, family planning and child development clinics are now fairly widespread but hypertension and diabetes are probably the two commonest diseases to be supervised in this way. The 1990 GP Contract, which includes payment for health promotion and disease management sessions has considerably stimulated clinic development.

The advantages of such sessions are that it enables different professionals such as doctors, nurses and dietitians to work together and helps to concentrate minds on what needs to be done. The number of clinics is likely to increase still further since they will attract extra remuneration in the 1990 GP Contract.

Practice managers clearly need to be involved in the setting up of these clinics and should be able to supply figures for planning purposes. The

EPILEPSY

> Patient's label

History (with dates):

Type of seizure:

Occupation:

Investigations/second opinion:

Counselling (enter dates):

Nature of disease:	Employment:
Trigger factors: (including alcohol)	Drug instructions: (including contraception)
First aid during a fit:	Free prescriptions:
Dangers of water/heights:	Inheritance/pregnancy:
Driving regulations:	British Epilepsy Association:

Drugs:

Problem list entered: Epilepsy: grand:mal / petit:mal / temporal:lobe / focal

Follow-up:

Date	No. fits since last review	Date last fit 'D' or 'N'	Comments (including work and social problems and drug levels if indicated)

Figure 14.1 Epilepsy flow sheet, Sonning Common Health Centre.

BP monitoring and assessment

Patient's label

Baseline readings

Date	Wt	BMI	BP	Comments	TCA

Other IHD risk factors

Family history	No	Yes	Overweight	No	Yes
Raised cholesterol	No	Yes	Diabetes	No	Yes
Smoking	Never		Stopped	Yes	

Further Details

Eng organ damage

Past history IHD	No	Yes	Raised creatinine	No	Yes
Fundi changes	No	Yes	Large heart (chest X-ray)	No	Yes
Proteinuria	No	Yes	LV hypertrophy (ECG)	No	Yes

Further details

Other hypotensive action

Weight reduction	No	Yes	Details
Salt reduction	No	Yes	Details
Limit alcohol (20u/pw)	No	Yes	Details

Further observation readings

Date	Wt	BMI	BP	Comments	TCA

Figure 14.2   Blood pressure assessment and monitoring sheet, Sonning Common Health Centre.

number of patients with the disorder and the average number of times they are seen each year will enable the demand to be calculated.

Use of hospital and related facilities

Unlike systems of health care in many other countries, the British tradition is that all patients have their own family doctor and, with one or two exceptions, patients only gain access to specialists and other professionals, such as physiotherapists, through their family doctor. There are considerable advantages in this system. It ensures that patients, when needing specialist care, go to the appropriate specialist: it protects patients from unnecessary specialist activity, and it allows specialists to devote their time to their particular field without having to see patients who do not need their services.

At the beginning of the NHS, GPs could not get direct access to diagnostic services and patients had to be referred to a specialist if they needed a blood test or X-ray. Today, the modern GP expects to diagnose and treat a large range of conditions with the help of the local pathology and X-ray departments with sophisticated investigations. Furthermore, many of the blood samples are taken in the practice now by one of the nurses and it is the blood, rather than the patient, that makes the journey to the laboratory.

Monitoring referrals

Under the 1990 GP Contract changes and others associated with the White Paper proposals practices need to monitor their use of some of the services provided for patients by external services.

The 1990 GP Contract requires annual reports to be submitted to the FHSA or Health Board which includes the number of hospital referrals both for in-patients and out-patients and use of diagnostic services. The exact list is shown in Table 14.9. Special forms will be issued.

Table 14.9   Annual reports for use of hospital services.

Number of hospital referrals (by clinical speciality) as
   (a)   in-patients
   (b)   out-patients
Number of direct referrals for hospital treatment
Use made of hospital diagnostic services
Number of self-referrals by patients where known

Source: *Health Departments of Great Britain: The 1990 Contract.*

The White Paper proposals for the future of the NHS[10] are based on a system of budgeting. Large practices (with lists of over 9000) are able to apply to hold their own budgets. As well as covering staff costs, premises, finance and prescribing costs these budgets will also cover the cost of out-patient referrals, diagnostic requests, certain forms of treatment and some in-patient costs. Other practices (the majority) will have budgets held on their behalf by the Health Authority.

Whilst practices holding their own budgets are involved in a major management and accounting exercise, all practices are now faced with needing to monitor their use of hospital and diagnostic services.

It is known from previous research[11] that GPs vary widely in all these areas. The percentage of patients they refer to consultants, the number of tests they order and the number of prescriptions they write are remarkably different and these variations are largely unexplained. Practice managers will have to set up systems to record the data required for the 1990 GP Contract and will subsequently need to provide running totals doctor by doctor so that problems of possible overspending can be anticipated. Clearly the easiest way of producing this information will be by computer but current systems do not generally have these facilities as yet.

Patient participation

During the last two decades there has been considerable debate about the nature of doctor–patient communication and ways in which patients can play a larger part in the decisions about their health care. In the Oxford Region much of the teaching for trainee GPs in communication skills in the consultation is based on the belief that what the patient contributes to the consultation is crucial[12].

This development has been mirrored by developments outside the consultation which has been described as patient participation, and in the early seventies three practices set up patient participation groups at Aberdare, Berinsfield and Bristol[13]. These have been followed by others and by 1978, 19 were known to be in operation[14].

Function

Pritchard has described the development of patient participation groups[15,16] and lists four main functions they seem to fulfil. First, they provide feedback for planning and evaluation. They should be a means by which doctors, nurses and practice managers can find out what patients want and are particularly relevant now that practices are having to make themselves more consumer orientated as described earlier in this chapter. It enables practices to sound out how far patients believe doctors and nurses should be probing their life-styles with a view to preventing disease, and it reminds the primary health team of some of the problems that people face in their homes and at work.

Second, patient participation groups (PPGs) are a useful channel for health education and for some this is their main activity. Whilst doctors and nurses have their own ideas about what patients need, the patients themselves also have their own priorities and should be able to take charge of organizing the programme. There are now plenty of videotapes and patient literature which can be used.

Third, the group can act as a safety valve, if one is needed. Whilst it cannot deal with an individual complaint it can air areas where there may be general dissatisfaction. Experience has shown, however, that PPGs generate few complaints and obviously this may reflect the fact that a practice which sets up a PPG is likely to be consumer orientated in the first place. This forum in which general problems can be aired may work in both directions. Patients may want to raise difficulties of access but doctors too may be having difficulties of their own. A high percentage of patients not keeping appointments could be one example. A forum in which all can look at constructive solutions seems a logical way of handling these kinds of issues.

There is a potential danger: PPGs can be used to sanction decisions that the doctors wish to take. A powerful group of doctors could in theory get a compliant group of patients to approve a course of action which may be convenient for the doctors but less so for the patients and use this as a means of justifying what they want to do. On the whole, however, it appears that such anxieties are ill-founded.

Fourth, PPGs can act as a social support service. Some have identified and set up activities to support the elderly and handicapped. These schemes often help the helpers as much as the helped and a mechanism for members of the practice population to help each other seems a useful and productive community exercise.

Setting up a group

One of the problems that arises when setting up a group is to decide how members will be selected. Some practices, such as Berinsfield, have used local organizations such as the Women's Institute and Parish Council to nominate people. Others have annual elections or have mechanisms to ensure a cross-section of age and occupation. Obviously it is important to try to get as representative a group as possible. Graffy[17] has described how some groups operate and Table 14.10, listing typical issues discussed by PPGs, is taken from his paper.

Table 14.10 Typical issues discussed by patient participation groups.

Structural:
  Waiting/play areas
  Privacy while making appointments
  Wheelchair ramps
  Parking facilities
  Planning new health centre

Staff:
  Staffing levels
  What is hoped for in a new partner
    (for example, woman preferred)
  Staff roles
  Staff attitudes (complimentary as well as critical)

Organizational:
  Surgery hours (evening/Saturday mornings)
  Appointment system
  Night calls
  Use of intercom to call patients

Services:
  Preventive and screening programmes
  Marriage guidance counselling
  Chiropody
  Home visiting for the elderly
  Community-based social work
  Health visiting

Policy:
  Medical student training
  Social worker and health visitor training
  Videotapes for teaching
  Hospital referrals
  Drug policy (hypnotics and antibiotics)
  Research work

Source: Graffy, J.P. (1981)[17].

There is a National Association for Patient Participation in General Practice which exists to circulate information and to hold conferences and meetings.

Equipment

During the last 40 years there has been a steady increase in technology in medicine. In the early years of the NHS much of this development took place in hospital whilst general practice remained relatively undeveloped. Then, gradually, new developments began to affect primary health care so that a modern general practice today possesses a wide range of sophisticated equipment.

Part of the reason for this development is miniaturization and reduction in cost. In the same way that computers have become cheaper and smaller, whilst increasing in power, so some of the more sophisticated diagnostic equipment has followed the same course. Electrocardiographs or ECGs (machines which analyse the electrical activity of the heart), for example, are now much smaller and more compact than they used to be and small machines producing rapid estimations of blood sugar levels are cheap and commonplace.

Equipping general practice is a potential problem in the NHS since GPs receive no direct reimbursement for purchases, nor can they recoup their costs by passing on charges to the patient in the way that a private practice or business can. So those GPs who purchase expensive equipment suffer a loss of income. That issue has not been addressed by the Government in its 1990 GP Contract.

The only mechanism whereby doctors could obtain reimbursement for all equipment is through the expenses component of their income. Each year the tax returns of GPs are sampled and the average expenses calculated: the amount is then added to doctors' pay the following year to reimburse them. Under this system the low spending doctors benefit whilst the high spending ones lose out. If however, all doctors increased their spending on equipment the sum would find its way back into the system.

Diagnostics

Broadly speaking most clinical equipment falls into two groups: one for helping doctors to make diagnoses and the other for treatment.

All doctors possess their own personal diagnostic equipment for use in the surgery or at home. This includes a stethoscope, auroscope (for looking in ears), ophthalmoscope (for looking at eyes) and a thermometer. But there is now quite a large range of equipment that will normally be shared between several doctors and kept on the premises: some of this will require servicing or repair when it goes wrong. The practice manager therefore needs to be familiar with the arrangements for contracts and who to contact in case of problems.

A recent survey of practices in Devon and Cornwall[18] has demonstrated the large amount of equipment that some practices possess and some of the commoner items are shown in Table 14.11.

Table 14.11   Common diagnostic equipment.

Visual acuity charts
Peak flow meters
Urine analysis multisticks
Blood sugar sticks
Proctoscope
Electrocardiograph
Sonicaid
Microscope
Glucometer

Source: Bradley, N. & Watkins, S. (1989)[18].

Other equipment less commonly found were audiometers (for testing hearing), vitalographs (similar to peak flow meters for testing lung function) and sigmoidoscopes and colonoscopes (for looking into the large bowel).

Treatment

Table 14.12 shows a list of some of the commoner equipment for treatment also taken from the recent Devon and Cornwall survey[18].

Table 14.12   Common treatment equipment.

Minor operations kit
Intravenous fluid and giving set
Electric nebulizer
Resuscitation kit
Oxygen
Electrocautery equipment

Source: Bradley, N. & Watkins, S. (1989)[18].

Other less common equipment found in the survey included liquid nitrogen equipment (for freezing warts) and defibrillators (for dealing with cardiac arrest). The 1990 GP Contract is likely to stimulate the need for minor operation equipment since there is special payment for such procedures.

Health Equipment Bulletin News

This bulletin publishes evaluation of electromedical equipment—recent ones have looked at blood pressure recorders and ECGs. NHS doctors can obtain copies free via their local health authorities.

The future

The next likely development is a range of diagnostic equipment that will enable doctors to do blood tests in the surgery or at home with immediate results like the way that blood sugar readings can be done now. New miniature analysing equipment with disposable probes will enable practices to dispense with the laboratory for some routine tests. This may be an attractive option for the larger practices who choose to operate their own budgets because they will be able to reduce their laboratory costs.

Sterilizing equipment

It is important that all practices have adequate sterilizing equipment because of the danger of passing infection from one person to another on diagnostic equipment, such as vaginal speculae and nebulizer mouth pieces. Most practices still possess boiler sterilizers but some are now moving to autoclaves which enable much higher temperatures to be achieved. Practice managers should be familiar with the current procedures in force and should ensure that all equipment is regularly checked and serviced.

Ethical issues

Because doctors have access to information that is sometimes very personal and hold a privileged position in society, it is extremely important that they behave at all times in an appropriate manner. They are often involved in consultations and physical examinations of an intimate nature and the General Medical Council issues guidance to doctors and identifies a number of areas where experience has shown difficulties may arise[2].

Personal relationships

Doctors must not use their professional position to become emotionally or sexually involved with patients. Any doctor who thinks a situation might develop or may wish to have such a relationship is advised to stop looking after that patient.

Confidentiality

It is a long established rule that information given to a doctor in a professional consultation is strictly confidential and must not, with certain exceptions, be divulged to third parties. Patients must be able to tell their doctors what they believe their doctors need to know in the certainty that such information is secure. It is equally important that all practice staff who come into contact with clinical information regard it as strictly confidential, and most practices have staff contracts that specify that any breaches of confidence are grounds for instant dismissal.

The exceptions when confidence can be broken include written consent by the patient, the sharing of information with other doctors, nurses and professionals involved in the care of the patient, and notification of certain infectious diseases.

There are two areas which are of direct concern to practice staff. The first is requests for information about the health of a patient from organizations such as insurance companies, employers and solicitors. Here it is important that the patient's written permission is available before any report is sent. Furthermore, patients now have the right to see reports for insurance and related purposes and the practice staff should check the patient's wishes which should be enclosed with insurance company requests.

The second concerns medical records. It is now commonplace for those practices approved for postgraduate training to have some of their medical records inspected by visiting doctors as part of their approval process. Whilst the GMC advises that clinical information is normally only shared with doctors 'who participate in or assume responsibility for clinical management of the patient' the Council also accepts that training practice approval is a means whereby standards can be maintained or approved. Its advice is that patients of such practices should be told in practice brochures or waiting room notices that their records may be scrutinized in this way and that they have the right to object.

Other issues

Problems relating to advertising have been referred to earlier in this chapter. Whilst rules governing the identification of doctors in the media are less strict than they used to be, practice staff should refer all journalists to the doctors concerned and under no circumstances should attempt to deal with them themselves.

Certification

Doctors are frequently asked for their signature to support applications for such things as passports and shotguns. They are also required to issue medical certificates some of which are of a statutory nature and must be issued in accordance with the instructions. Medical certificates, like prescriptions, should be kept locked up and not left lying about.

Complaints

From time to time practices have to deal with patients who believe they are not getting the service to which they are entitled. One of the commonest causes of dissatisfaction is the inability of patients to see or speak to the doctor as soon as they believe they should.

All practice staff need to understand why patients may get angry and how to deal with these difficult situations. Many of them can be handled with understanding and tact and indeed if complaints are dealt with competently and sympathetically from the outset it is much less likely that they will escalate into greater problems.

Many of the patients attending the surgery are anxious and anger is often a symptom of anxiety. The important point for all staff is not to allow themselves to get angry too. If a difficult situation develops at the reception desk, the practice manager should invite the patient into her office so that the matter can be resolved away from the scrutiny of others in the waiting area. Equally, if a patient becomes demanding on the telephone the practice manager should take over. Whilst it is important to give the patient his or her say and to be helpful, outright rudeness to staff should not be tolerated and one of the doctors should be involved if difficulties continue.

Some problems can be handled by the practice manager. Clearly, however, if there is a suggestion that the patient's medical care has been unsatisfactory in some way, the patient's doctor must be involved immediately. Once again, as the Medical Defence Union puts it in its advice to doctors, 'care, communication and courtesy are all-important'.

Hopefully these situations will be few and far between. If the practice manager believes that the practice is getting more than its fair share of complaints she should take steps to find out why and discuss it with the doctors.

Conclusions

Many practice managers in the past have occupied limited roles being concerned chiefly with organizing staff rotas and making certain that the building is cleaned. It will have become clear from this book that the role of the modern practice manager is very much wider than that envisaged when such appointments were first made.

This chapter has endeavoured to emphasize that the practice manager has key responsibilities in patient care. Not only do these cover all matters to do with access but they should now be encompassing aspects of health promotion and beginning to move into auditing the management of disease itself.

Throughout its short history the primary health team has moved through various phases of development. In the sixties the emphasis was on attaching health visitors and district nurses from health authorities. In the seventies and eighties practice nurses came into their own. The nineties will be the decade of the practice manager.

References

1. Health Departments of Great Britain (1989) *General practice in the NHS. The 1990 Contract.*
2. General Medical Council (1987) *Professional conduct and discipline: fitness to practise.*
3. NHS Review (1989) *Indicative prescribing budgets for general medical practitioners.* Working Paper No. 4. HMSO, London.
4. Drury, V.W.M. (1989) Repeat prescribing: a review. *Journal of the Royal College of General Practitioners,* **32**, 42–45.
5. Pritchard, P.M.M., Low, K. & Whalen, M. (1984) *Management in general practice,* pp. 133–135, Oxford University Press.
6. Anderson, P. (1988) Excess mortality associated with alcohol consumption. *British Medical Journal,* **297**, 824–826.
7. Lawrence, M.S.T.A. (1988) All together now. *Journal of the Royal College of General Practitioners,* **38**, 296–302.
8. Fullard, E., Fowler, G.H. & Gray, J.M. (1984) Facilitating prevention in primary care. *British Medical Journal,* **289**, 1585–1587.
9. Schofield, T.P.C., Hasler, J.C. & Barnes, G. (1990) Implications for practice. In: J.C. Hasler & T.P.C. Schofield (eds) *Continuing Care: the management of chronic disease,* 2nd edn, Oxford University Press.
10. Secretaries of State for Health; England, Wales, Northern Ireland and Scotland (1989) *Working for patients.* HMSO, London.
11. Metcalfe, D. (1986) Variations in process in primary care. In: D.A. Pendleton, T.P.C. Schofield & M. Marinker (eds) *In Pursuit of Quality.* pp. 96–110. Royal College of General Practitioners, London.
12. Pendleton, D.A. *et al.* (1984) *The consultation. An approach to learning and teaching.* Oxford University Press.

13. Dakin, A. & Mulligan, J. (1980) Patient participation. *Journal of the Royal College of General Practitioners*, **30**, 133–135.
14. Mant, J. (1978) *Gazeteer of patient participation groups.* Central Information Service for General Medical Practice, London.
15. Pritchard, P. (ed.) (1981) *Patient participation in general practice.* Royal College of General Practitioners, Occasional Paper No. 17.
16. Pritchard, P.M.M. (1983) Patient participation. In: D.A. Pendleton & J.C. Hasler (eds) *Doctor–patient communication.* pp. 205–221. Academic Press, London.
17. Graffy, J.P. (1981) Patient participation in primary health care. In: P. Pritchard (ed.) *Patient participation in general practice.* Royal College of General Practitioners, Occasional Paper No. 17.
18. Bradley, N. & Watkins, S. (1989) Survey of equipment in general practice. *British Medical Journal*, **299**, 435–436.

Index

absenteeism 73
accessibility 203–7
accident book 115
accidents 11, 112, 115
accountants 153
  duties 167
  fees 166–7
  role of 165–7
accounting procedures 153–9
accounts
  in a fund-holding practice 195–6,
    196–7
  reading 169–80
activity analyses 121–3
acute illness 2
administration 32–4
administration charge, in fund-holding
    practice 193
advertisements
  job 55–7
  for the practice 202
age discrimination 54
age-sex register 211–12
aged, services to 11
AHCPA 20
aims 22–3
alcohol abuse 74
  by doctors 47–8
AMSPAR 20
antenatal care, time off for 66
application forms 57
appointment schedules 204
Association of Health Centre and Practice
    Administrations 20
Association of Medical Secretaries, Practice
    Administrators and Receptionists 20
audit
  of communications 85
  cycle 133
  medical 130–3
  of the practice 134–6
availability 203–7
awareness of change outside work 31–2

Basic Practice Allowance 144
behavioural psychology 83
BMA 11
  as contact for sick doctors 48
body language 86–7
bookkeeping 153–9
BPA 144

budget 27–8, 153–5
  formulation in fund-holding
    practices 192–3
  monitoring performance against 31
business plans 195

capitation fees 145
certification of confinement 79
certification 228–9
cervical cytology programme 9
  fees 146
CHCs 12–13
Child Health Surveillance Programme 9
  fees for 145
chronic disease 2–3, 216–17
  clinics 218, 221
  protocols 217–18
  records 281, 219–20
clinics 218, 221
collected data audit 135–6
Commission for Racial Equality 78
communication 85
  auditing 90–2
  clarity 87–8
  inter-personal 86–9
  non-verbal 86–7
  systems 89–92
Community Health Councils 12–13
comparability 125–6
competition 200
complaints 8, 46–7, 229
compliance, securing 29–30
computers 34
  establishing priorities 26–7
  in patient registration 212
  in prescribing 210
  systems in fund-holding practices 197
confidentiality 228
constructive dismissal 76
consultations, length of 13
continuing education 20
continuity of care 2–3
contract of employment 58–60
  frustration of 76
  repudiation 76
  termination 75–6
  varying 74
controlled drugs 208
COSHH regulations 113
cost-effectiveness 134
cost-rent schemes 168–9
  limits 186

councillors, right to time off 68
County Court 78
critical event audit 131–3, 134–5
custom and practice 59

deductions 59
Dead of Partnership 40–1
delegation 138–9
DHA 9–10
diagnostic equipment 225–6
diagnostic services 221
'direct discrimination' 53–4
disabled people, employment of 52–3
disciplinary penalties 70–2
disciplinary procedure 69–70
disciplinary rules 68–9
disease index 212–13
disease prevention 3–4, 213–16
dismissal 71–3
  constructive 76
dispensing 208
  fees 148
District Health Authority 9–10
district nurses 49
drawings systems 158–62, 163
drug abuse 74
  by doctors 47–8
drugs
  categories 208
  dispensing 148, 208
  information 207
  safeguards 208

elderly, services to 11
employee development 64
employer-determined conditions 59
employment law 51–82
employment protection 76–8
Employment Protection (Consolidation)
    Act 1978 60–1
employment status 55
Equal Opportunities Commission 78
equal pay 64–5
equalized drawings systems 161–2, 163
equipment 225–7
ethics 227–9
expenditure levels 181

family care 1–2
Family Health Services Authority
    (FHSA) 7–9
  consultation with LMCs 10
  and fund-holding initiative 191
  views on quality of care 119–20
Family Practitioner Committee (FPC) 7
  fees and allowances 143–4, 184–5
FHSA see Family Health Services Authority

final written warning 71
financial management 138–86
financial plan 27
financial targets 23
flexible approach, importance of 25
formal verbal warning 71
FPC 7
fund-holding initiative 191–8, 222

General Medical Services Committee 11
general practice
  changes in 13–14
  nature 1–5
  structure and external
    relationships 6–13
general practitioner (GP)
  job definition 5
  numbers of 13
  relationship with health service 6–7
  relationship with practice
    manager 38–48
  views on quality of service 118–19
generic prescribing 187, 207
GP Fund-holder's manual of
    accounts 195–6
group dynamics 103
group practice, advantages of 13

health and safety 109
  action list 115–16
  employees' responsibilities 113–14
  employer's duties 109–12
  law enforcement 114–15
  written policy 110–11
Health and Safety at Work Act 1974 110
Health and Safety Executive
    inspectors 109, 114–15
health centres 168
health education 213–14
Health Equipment Bulletin News 227
health promotion 3–4, 213–16
  fees for 146
health visitors 49
home visits 205
hospital referrals 196, 221–2
hospital staff, views on quality of
    care 119
HSE inspectors 109, 114–15

ill health, absence from work due to 73–4
IMA 189
immunization 214–15
  fees 146
implied terms 59–60
income generation
  NHS 144–7
  non-NHS 147–9

income tax   82, 142
    reserve accounts   164–5
independent contractor status   6–7
    advantages   140–2
    disadvantages   142
independent medical adviser   189
indicative prescribing amounts   189–90,
    209
'indirect discrimination'   54–5
induction
    checklist   17–19
    importance   15–16
    after promotion   19
    responsibility for   19–20
    timing   16–17
Industrial Tribunal   55, 72, 74, 76–8
informal verbal warning   70–1
internal control questionnaire   149–51
interviews   16, 57–8
item-of-service fees   146, 181–2

job advertisements   55–7
job description   48–9, 52
job evaluation   31
job share   55
job title   56

language proficiency   55
leave advances   149
local authorities   11–12
Local Health Committees (LHCs)   12
Local Medical Committees
    (LMCs)   10–11

magistrates, right to time off   68
management   21–32
    structure, under fund-holding
        initiative   194–5
Manual of accounts   195–6
Maslow's Theory of Human
    Motivation   93–4
maternity leave   66, 79–80
maternity pay   67, 80–1
medical audit
    attitudes to   130–1
    definition   130
    resources   131
    types   131–3
Medical Audit Advisory Groups   10
medical records see patient records
medical students, allowances for   147
MIMS   207
minor surgery fees   147
monitoring performance   30–1
motivation   92–102
    and team balance   103–4

National Insurance   81, 162–4
negotiated agreements   59
NHS, structure   8
night visit fees   146
non-verbal communication   86–7
notice   75
    and dismissal   71
noticeboards   90
nurse facilitator   216

objectives, establishing   22–3, 99–102,
    199
Occupier's Liability Act 1957   112
offer of appointment   58
office organization   89–90
opportunistic screening   215–16
OTC drugs   208
outgoings, control of   151–2
over the counter drugs   208
overspending   198

PACT system   187–8, 209
partnership agreements   39–41
patient records   216
    in chronic disease   218, 219–20
    confidentiality   228
patients
    impact of administration on   33–4
    information for   214
    new, routine consultation with   202
    participation groups   222–4
    questionnaires to   123
    registration   211
    satisfaction   117
pay statements   61
PAYE   82
    see also income tax
pensions   141
performance appraisal   49, 63–4,
    94–102, 137
performance monitoring   30–1
person specification   52, 53
personal relationships   227
personality conflicts   45–6
personnel management   51–82
petty cash   154–8
pharmaceutical company
    representatives   209
policies, practice   90
'positive action'   55, 56, 64
postgraduate education allowance   145
practice allowances   144
practice boundaries   205–7
practice budget   27–8, 153–5
    formulation in fund-holding
        practices   192–3
    monitoring performance against   31

practice data, presentation and
    assessment   127–8
practice image   200–1
practice leaflets   200, 201
practice manager   229–30
    administrative role   32–4
    comparison with managers in
        industry   34–6
    contact with outside world   31–2
    disciplinary responsibilities   72
    as financial controller   138–9
    and induction training   19–20
    interface with doctors   38–48
    interface with office staff   48–9
    interface with other staff   49
    management role   21–32
    role of   37–50
Practice Manager Development
    Programme   64
practice meetings   41–4
practice nurse   49
Practice Receptionist Programme   64
practice reports   128–9
practice staff   14
    continuing education   20
    recruitment   51–62
    view of quality of care   118
    see also training
pregnancy, employment rights
    during   66–7
premises   167–9
    accessibility   204
prescribing   187–90
    audit   121, 123, 124, 209
    budgets   189–90, 209
    computerized   210
    generic   187, 207
    repeat   209–10
preventive medicine   3–4, 213–16
primary care   1
    see also general practice
primary health care team   104
priorities, establishing   25–7
private work, fees for   154
'pro-active' work patterns   3–4
procedures   90
    defining   23–5
    need for   33–4
    notes of   89
profitability, ensuring   139–40
promoting the practice   199–202
promotion   64
    induction training following   19

qualifications   55
quality
    defining   117

measurement   120–3
    and standards   123–8
    views on   117–20
questionnaires, patient   123

racial discrimination   53–4
Radcliffe Medical Press, courses run by   20
random case analysis   120
'reactive' work patterns   3–4
receptionists   201, 202
record review   121
recruitment   51–62
Red Book   10, 143–4, 182
referrals   196, 221–2
refunds   148–9
Regional Health Authority   9
    and fund-holding initiative   191
registration fees   145
repeat prescriptions   209–10
    computerization   210
resources, securing and allocating   27–8
retirement age   67
Review Body   143
rights to time off   67–8
roles, defining   23–5
rotas   45
rules   33

safety committees   112
safety policy, written statement
    of   110–11
safety representatives   111–12
sampling   124–5
score grids   121, 122
screening   215–16
secondary care   1
secondary groups   103
self-audit   84–5
self-employment   141–3
self-governing units   11
senior partner, disciplinary
    responsibilities   71
senior receptionist, disciplinary
    responsibilities   72
seniority payments   145
sessional fees   146–7
sex discrimination   53–4
sickness absences   73–4, 78–9
'small within large' organization   34
SMP   67, 80–1
social functions   108
Social Services Department, relationship
    with general practice   11–12
social workers   49
    attachment to practices   12

SSP 78–9
staff meetings 49
staff recruitment 51–62
standardization 126–7
standardized protocols 123
standards 123–8
Statement of fees and allowances see
    Red Book
statement of terms and conditions 60–2
statistics 181–2
Statutory Maternity Pay 67, 80–1
Statutory Sick Pay 78–9
sterilizing equipment 227
suggestion box technique 107
summary dismissal 71
superannuation 141
supervisory style 29–30
surgery premises 167–9

tasks, defining 23–5
teamwork 103–7, 216
time management 28
time off, rights to 67–8
trade union representatives, right to time
    off 67–8

training 15–20, 49, 64
    in communication skills 88–9
    finding time for 84
    need for 84
    policy 102
training practices 13
treatment equipment 226

underspending 198
unfair dismissal 72–3

verbal warnings 70–1

waiting room 201
waiting time audit 135–6
weekly timetable 28
wholism 4
women, age discrimination against 54
'word of mouth' recruitment 56–7
Working for patients 119, 130, 191
workload monitoring 204
written warning 71